C-EFM® EXAM PREP
STUDY GUIDE

C-EFM® EXAM PREP STUDY GUIDE

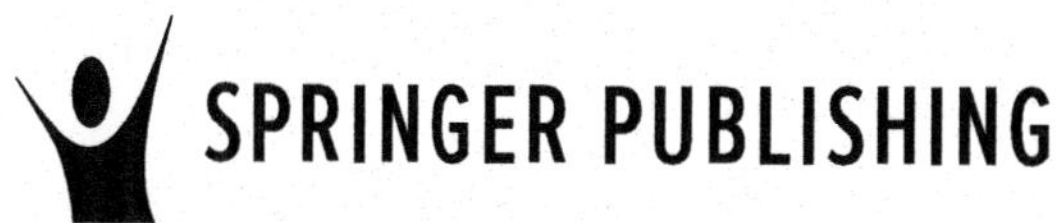

Springer Publishing Company, LLC
11 West 42nd Street, New York, NY 10036
www.springerpub.com

Acquisitions Editor: Jaclyn Koshofer
Compositor: Exeter Premedia Services Private Ltd.

ISBN: 978-0-8261-6575-6
ebook ISBN: 978-0-8261-6625-8
DOI: 10.1891/ 9780826166258

24 25 26 / 5 4 3 2

The author and the publisher of this Work have made every effort to use sources believed to be reliable to provide information that is accurate and compatible with the standards generally accepted at the time of publication. The author and publisher shall not be liable for any special, consequential, or exemplary damages resulting, in whole or in part, from the readers' use of, or reliance on, the information contained in this book. The publisher has no responsibility for the persistence or accuracy of URLs for external or third-party Internet websites referred to in this publication and does not guarantee that any content on such websites is, or will remain, accurate or appropriate.

C-EFM® is a registered trademark of National Certification Corporation (NCC). NCC does not endorse this resource, nor does it have a proprietary relationship with Springer Publishing Company.

Library of Congress Control Number: 2023930030

Contact sales@springerpub.com to receive discount rates on bulk purchases.

Publisher's Note: New and used products purchased from third-party sellers are not guaranteed for quality, authenticity, or access to any included digital components.

Printed in the United States of America by Gasch Printing.

CONTENTS

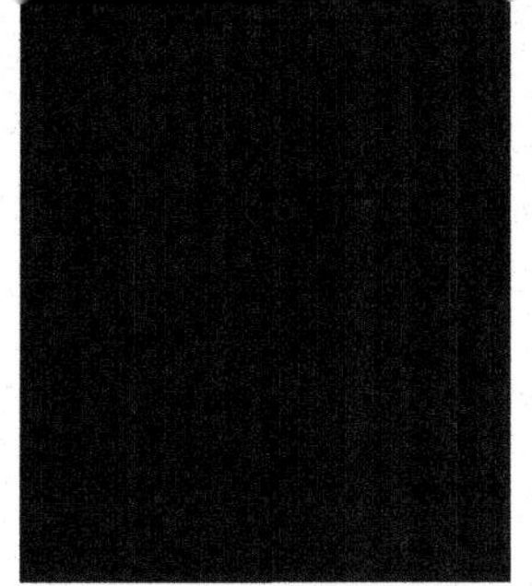

PREFACE

This *Exam Prep Study Guide* was designed to be a high-speed review—a last-minute gut check before your exam day. We created this review to supplement to your certification preparation studies. We encourage you to use it in conjunction with other study aids to ensure you are as prepared as possible for the exam.

This book follows the National Certification Corporation's most recent exam content outlines and uses a succinct, bulleted format to highlight what you need to know. The aim of this book is to help you solidify your retention of information in the month or so leading up to your exam. It is written by certified practitioners who are familiar with the exam and the content you need to know. Special features appear throughout the book to call out important information, including:

- **Complications**: Problems that can arise with certain disease states or procedures
- **Nursing Pearls**: Additional patient care insights and strategies for knowledge retention
- **Alerts**: Need-to-know details on how to handle emergency situations or when to transfer care
- **Pop Quizzes**: Critical-thinking questions to test your ability to synthesize what you learned (answers in the back of the book)
- **Two Full-Length Practice Tests**: One printed in the book, one online
- **Free One-Month Access to ExamPrepConnect**: The digital study platform that guides you confidently through your exam prep journey

We know life is busy. Being able to prepare for your exam efficiently and effectively is paramount, which is why we created this *Exam Prep Study Guide*. You have come to the right place as you continue on your path of professional growth and development. The stakes are high, and we want to help you succeed. Best of luck to you on your certification journey.

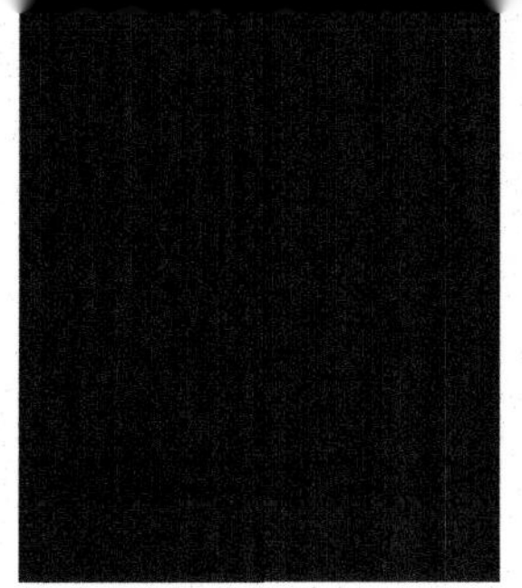

PASS GUARANTEE

If you use this resource to prepare for your exam and do not pass, you may return it for a refund of your full purchase price, excluding tax, shipping, and handling. To receive a refund, return your product along with a copy of your exam score report and original receipt showing purchase of new product (not used). Product must be returned and received within 180 days of the original purchase date. Refunds will be issued within 8 weeks from acceptance and approval. One offer per person and address. This offer is valid for U.S. residents only. Void where prohibited. To initiate a refund, please contact Customer Service at csexamprep@springerpub.com.

1 GENERAL EXAMINATION INFORMATION

OVERVIEW

- The National Certification Corporation, founded in 1975 as a not-for-profit organization, offers multiple specialty certifications, including the subspecialty certification in electronic fetal monitoring (EFM). EFM is a tool that provides the bedside clinician with real-time data concerning the status of both the pregnant patient and the fetus. Safety and quality of inpatient care are central to the mission of healthcare institutions, and EFM-certified healthcare professionals show commitment to their education and expertise and to providing optimal care.

CERTIFICATION REQUIREMENTS

- C-EFM® applicants must hold current, active, and unencumbered licensure in the United States or Canada as a physician, RN, nurse practitioner, nurse midwife or midwife, physician assistant, or paramedic.

ABOUT THE EXAMINATION

- This certification is offered via computer at a computer test center or at home with live remote proctoring.
- The National Certification Corporation provides a content outline for the C-EFM examination on its website that includes the percentage distribution of questions per each major content category. This is included as part of the National Certification Corporation Candidate Guide: Electronic Fetal Monitoring C-EFM®, which is updated annually.
- The 2-hour computer-based certification examination contains up to 125 test questions; 100 of the questions are scored and the other 25 questions are included as pretest items. The pretest items do not impact the final score of the assessment. All questions are multiple choice with a premise and three possible answers.
- The 125 questions are broken down into the following categories: electronic monitoring equipment (5%); physiology (11%); pattern recognition and intervention (70%); fetal assessment methods (9%); professional issues (5%).

HOW TO APPLY

- Applications for the exam are accepted online only on the National Certification Corporation website. The National Certification Corporation sends application confirmation via email, and it can take from 1 to 14 days to process, review, and approve applications.
- Once approved, applicants have 90 days from the date of the application to take the exam and must schedule the exam within the first 30 days of the eligibility window.
- The exam cost is $210, including a $50 application fee.

HOW TO RECERTIFY

The National Certification Corporation certification must be maintained every 3 years. Certification that is not maintained will expire. The National Certification Corporation certification maintenance program allows certification holders to continue certification status by obtaining 15 hours of continuing education credit. For continuing education credit to be used for certification maintenance, it must be earned between the date of notification of certification and the date maintenance is due.

HOW TO CONTACT NATIONAL CERTIFICATION CORPORATION

Website: nccwebsite.org
Email address: info@nccnet.org

Mailing address:
National Certification Corporation
676 N. Michigan Avenue, Suite 3600
Chicago, IL 60611

MATERNAL–FETAL OXYGENATION: PHYSIOLOGY AND PATHOPHYSIOLOGY

MATERNAL–FETAL OXYGENATION

- Fetal oxygenation collectively depends on adequate maternal oxygenation; a healthy, functioning placenta; adequate maternal blood flow and volume; and adequate umbilical circulation.
- Three phases of oxygenation must occur to oxygenate the fetus: There must be adequate oxygenation of the pregnant patient. The patient must pass oxygenated blood to the placenta; at the placenta, satisfactory gas exchange must occur. The oxygenated blood is then transferred to the fetus via the umbilical cord.
- Fetal circulation: As described earlier, oxygen-rich blood flows from maternal circulation to fetal circulation via the placenta to the umbilical cord. The umbilical vein passes through the fetal liver and then splits. Most of the oxygenated blood passes through a shunt, the ductus venosus, where it is taken to the inferior vena cava and then enters the right side of the fetal heart (Figure 2.1). ▶

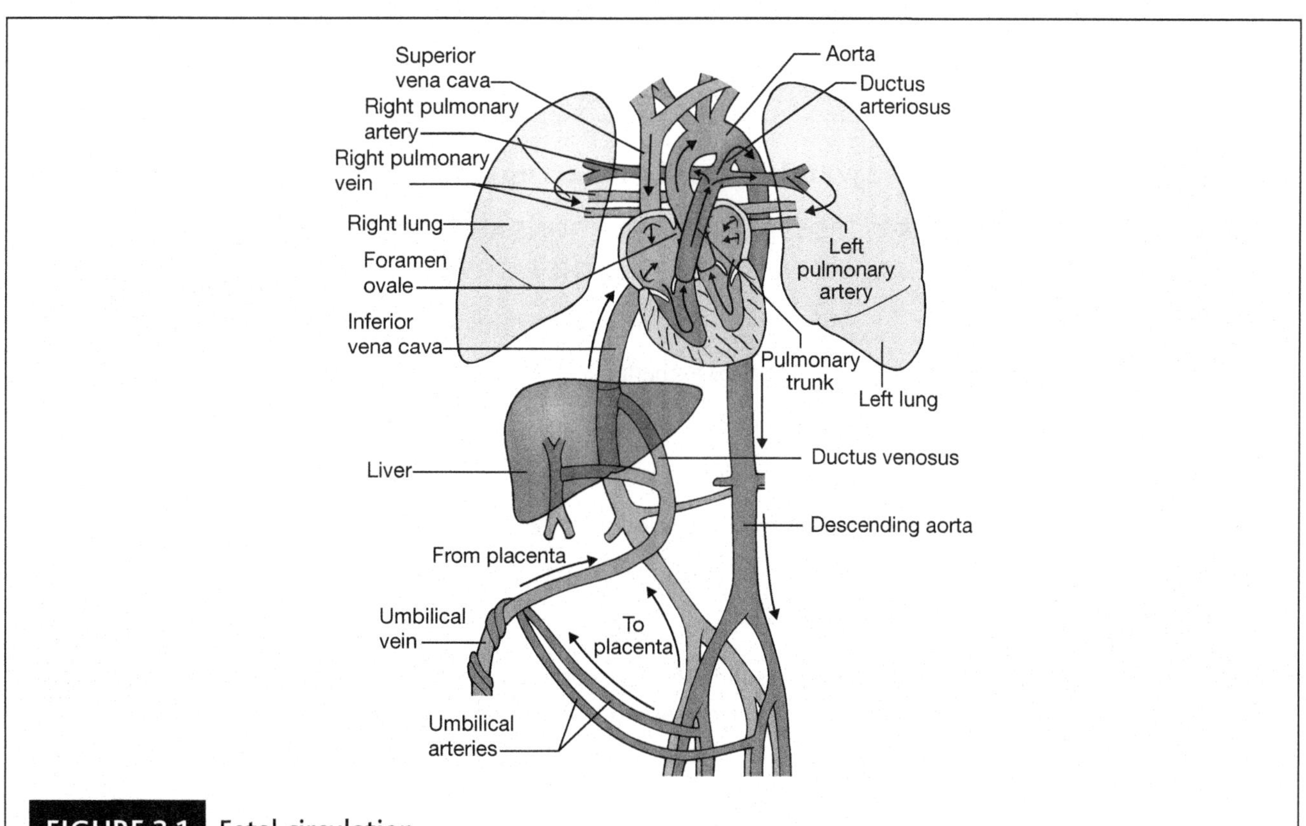

FIGURE 2.1 Fetal circulation.

Source: Jnah, A. J., & Trembath, A. N. (2018). *Fetal and neonatal physiology for the advanced practice nurse.* Springer Publishing Company.

MATERNAL–FETAL OXYGENATION (*continued*)

- Fetal heart: Oxygen-rich blood flows through one of the two connections in the fetal heart—the foramen ovale and the ductus arteriosus. The foramen ovale allows oxygen-rich blood to go from the right atrium to the left atrium, and then to the left ventricle and out the aorta to the brain. The blood circulates through the brain and arms, and then returns to the right atrium through the superior vena cava. Very little of this blood mixes with the oxygenated blood. This blood then enters the right ventricle. The less oxygenated blood leaves the right ventricle through the aorta, where a small amount travels to the lungs. The rest of the blood is shunted through the ductus arteriosus to the descending aorta. This allows for oxygen-poor blood to leave the fetus through the umbilical cord arteries and return to the placenta to receive oxygen.
- Oxygen follows the steps in the maternal–fetal pathway to transfer from the environment, through the maternal body systems and essential organs, to the fetus. There can be interruptions at any step along the pathway, affecting fetal oxygenation (Table 2.1).

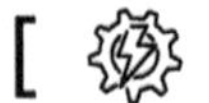 **ALERT!**

Once the oxygenated blood is delivered to the fetus, the blood enters the fetal circulation.

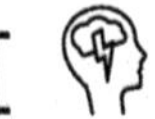 **COMPLICATIONS**

Interruptions of normal oxygen transfer can occur at any point along the maternal–fetal oxygenation pathway and cause fetal distress or demise.

 **POP QUIZ 2.1**

What interventions can be implemented by the nurse to improve uteroplacental circulation?

TABLE 2.1 Oxygen Pathway and Possible Interruptions	
STEPS FOR OXYGEN TRANSFER FROM ENVIRONMENT TO FETUS	**POSSIBLE INTERRUPTIONS AFFECTING FETAL OXYGENATION AT EACH POINT ON THE PATHWAY**
1. Environmental conditions	Alteration in normal maternal respirations of 21% oxygenated air
2. Maternal respiratory system	Impaired gas exchange
3. Maternal blood flow	Decreased cardiac output
4. Maternal vasculature	Impaired blood flow
5. Uterus	Uterine contractions or injury
6. Placenta	Disruption of maternal/fetal gas exchange
7. Umbilical cord	Compression or injury
8. Fetus	Fetal response to interruptions in the oxygen pathway includes consequences such as hypoxia and fetal injury

RESOURCES

Ahmed, W. A. S., & Hamdy, M. A. (2018). Optimal management of umbilical cord prolapse. *International Journal of Women's Health, 10*, 459–465. https://doi.org/10.2147/IJWH.S130879

American College of Obstetricians and Gynecologists. (2020). Gestational hypertension and preeclampsia. *Obstetrics & Gynecology, 135*(6), e237–e260. https://doi.org/10.1097/aog.0000000000003891

American Pregnancy Association. (2021). *Umbilical cord prolapse and compression.* https://americanpregnancy.org/healthy-pregnancy/pregnancy-complications/umbilical-cord-prolapse

Castillo-Castrejon, M., & Powell, T. L. (2017). Placental nutrient transport in gestational diabetic pregnancies. *Frontiers in Endocrinology, 8*, Article 306. https://doi.org/10.3389/fendo.2017.00306

Children's Hospital of Philadelphia. (2014). *Blood circulation in the fetus and newborn.* https://www.chop.edu/conditions-diseases/blood-circulation-fetus-and-newborn

Kawakita, T., Huang, C. C., & Landy, H. J. (2018). Risk factors for umbilical cord prolapse at the time of artificial rupture of membranes. *AJP Reports, 8*(2), e89–e94. https://doi.org/10.1055/s-0038-1649486

Mayo Clinic. (2021). *Preeclampsia.* https://www.mayoclinic.org/diseases-conditions/preeclampsia/symptoms-causes/syc-20355745

Miller, L. A., Miller, D. A., & Cypher, R. L. (2017). *Mosby's pocket guide to fetal monitoring: A multidisciplinary approach* (8th ed.). Elsevier.

Murray, M., Huelsmann, G., & Koperski, N. (2019). *Essentials of fetal and uterine monitoring* (5th ed.). Springer Publishing Company.

Nye, R. (2019). *Essentials of fetal heart rate monitoring* (chap. 7). Springer Publishing Company.

Prescribers' Digital Reference. (2022). *Invanz* [Drug information]. https://www.pdr.net/drug-information/invanz?druglabelid=359

Sholapurkar, S. L. (2019). Myths at the core of intrapartum cardiotocography interpretation—Risks of false ideology, prospect theory and way forward. *Clinical Obstetrics, Gynecology and Reproductive Medicine, 5*, 1–9. https://doi.org/10.15761/COGRM.1000253

3 MONITORING EQUIPMENT AND ASSESSMENT METHODS

ELECTRONIC FETAL MONITORING

Overview

- Electronic fetal monitoring (EFM) is a tool that provides the bedside clinician with real-time data regarding the status of both the patient and the fetus.
- EFM uses internal monitors, external monitors, or a combination to measure and record the heart rate of the fetus as well as the pattern of the patient's uterine contractions.
- A printout of the monitored data is known as the *EFM tracing*.

Sample Tracing Strip

Figure 3.1 explains the components of a sample EFM strip.

ELECTRONIC FETAL MONITORING EQUIPMENT

Overview

- Fetal heart monitoring is a vital part of caring for a patient in labor. The RN must understand when, why, and how fetal monitoring equipment is used. Fetal monitoring equipment is important, but it is used *in addition to* the nurse's assessment, not as a replacement for a nurse assessment. ▶

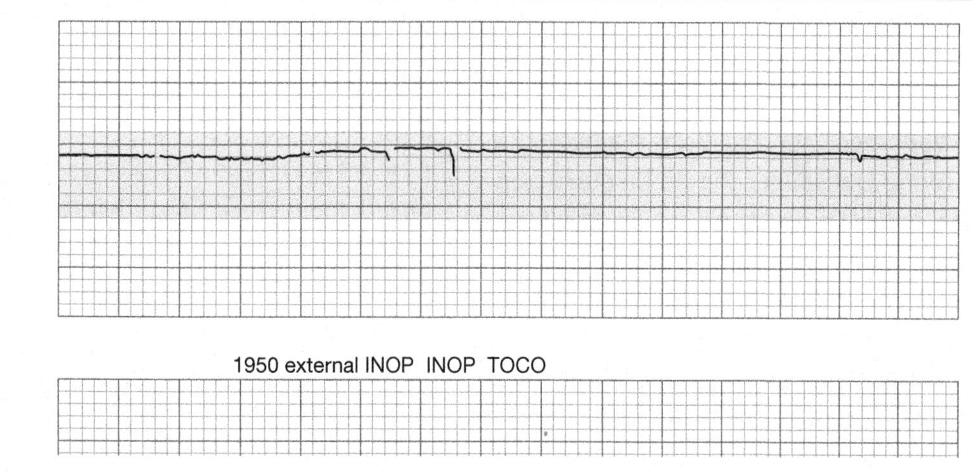

FIGURE 3.1 Sample tracing strip. The intervals between the vertical lines represent 1 minute of monitoring. The fetal heart rate tracing is displayed in the upper pane, and uterine activity is displayed in the lower pane.

Source: Nye, R. (2019). *Essentials of fetal heart rate monitoring.* Springer Publishing Company.

Overview (*continued*)

- Routine use of *continuous* fetal monitoring is not recommended for low-risk patients; however, *intermittent* fetal monitoring is appropriate for low-risk patients.
- Continuous fetal monitoring is considered appropriate for high-risk patients. Diagnoses considered at high risk include maternal diabetes, fetal defects, maternal cardiac conditions, and preeclampsia.
- There are two categories of EFM equipment: external monitoring, using an ultrasound transducer, and internal monitoring, using a fetal scalp electrode (FSE).
- There are two categories of potential issues with fetal monitoring equipment: artifact and equipment failure.

External Monitoring

- External monitoring typically requires patients to be physically connected to a monitor, which limits movement in labor. Some monitors offer wireless devices that can allow for movement, but these are not available in all facilities.
- Doppler ultrasound transducer: A monitor is placed on the patient's abdomen to continuously monitor fetal heart rate (FHR). The ultrasound transducer sends sound waves and records the echoing waves of the FHR.
- Fetoscope: A fetoscope is a type of stethoscope that is used to listen to, or auscultate, the FHR. Place the fetoscope on the patient's abdomen to listen for the fetal heartbeat. Count the FHR by using a timer or a watch or clock with a second hand. FHR is calculated in beats per minute (bpm).
- Tocodynamometer: A tocodynamometer is a pressure-sensitive device placed on the patient's abdomen over the uterus to measure uterine contractions. It measures only when contractions occur and how long they last; their strength must be palpated. It does not measure FHR, but it is required to determine the relationship between FHR and contractions.

Nursing Interventions

- Use Leopold's maneuver to locate the back of the fetus and place the ultrasound transducer on the patient's abdomen. For the best reading, the Doppler ultrasound transducer should be placed on the side of the patient's abdomen where the fetal back is located.
- Move the transducer around the patient's abdomen until the FHR is heard the most loudly.
- If the FHR cannot be found, ask the patient where the FHR is normally found, or request bedside ultrasound by the OB provider to confirm location and presence of FHR.
- Use a band or strap to hold the ultrasound transducer in place.
- Place the tocodynamometer on the patient's fundus, where the contractions are most intense; it may need to be moved when the patient repositions.
- Document FHR assessment, any interventions, and patient response per facility policy.

[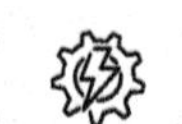]   **ALERT!**

A benefit of EFM is detection of early fetal distress resulting from fetal hypoxia and metabolic acidosis. Continuous fetal monitoring has been used to determine hypoxic-ischemic encephalopathy, cerebral palsy, and impending fetal death during labor. However, these events have a low prevalence, and continuous EFM has a false-positive rate of 99% in low-risk patients, which has been shown to increase the risk of Cesarean section.

[ ] **POP QUIZ 3.1**

A patient requires an external monitoring device. The nurse cannot locate the FHR after moving the transducer around. The patient shows the nurse where the FHR is usually heard, but the nurse still cannot locate it. What should the nurse do next?

Internal Monitoring

- Internal monitors are inserted through a dilated cervix.
- Membranes must be ruptured in order to use an internal monitoring device.
- Patient movement is limited when connected to the monitor.
- Types of internal monitoring devices include: FSE—an electrode inserted vaginally onto the fetal scalp that measures FHR. It must be inserted by a skilled provider. Intrauterine pressure catheter (IUPC)—a catheter placed in the uterus to measure uterine contraction frequency, duration, strength, and resting tone. Using the IUPC is the only way to accurately measure strength of contractions using Montevideo units.

Nursing Interventions

- Assist provider with equipment for FSE or IUPC.
- Assess and document, per institutional policy, the patient's heart rate, the FHR, any interventions, and the patient response.
- Follow and perform FHR assessments according to recommendations from professional organizations (including American College of Obstetricians and Gynecologists [ACOG] and Association of Women's Health, Obstetric and Neonatal Nurses [AWHONN]): low-risk patient—every 15 to 30 minutes in labor, every 5 to 15 minutes while pushing; high-risk patient—every 15 minutes in labor, every 5 minutes while pushing.

Artifact

- Artifact occurs when there is a signal processing error. The fetal heart monitor recognizes and traces the patient's heart rate, not the FHR.
- Accelerations during pushing indicate that the fetal heart monitor is recognizing the patient's heart rate, not the FHR (Figure 3.2).
- FHR monitors have built-in autocorrelation algorithms that enable them to create a smooth FHR tracing.
- FHR may be absent due to fetal demise, so the FHR monitor may display the patient's heart rate instead.

Nursing Interventions

- Confirm fetal life before EFM with a bedside ultrasound.
- Measure the patient's pulse by continuous pulse oximetry while monitoring FHR.

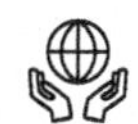

NURSING PEARL

The strength of contractions is calculated by internally (not externally) measuring peak uterine pressure amplitude in mmHg, subtracting the resting tone of the contraction, and adding up the numbers in a 10-minute period. The peak resting tone × number of contractions in 10 minutes = x mmHg (Montevideo units).

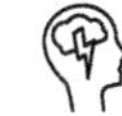

COMPLICATIONS

Because they require the amniotic sac to be broken, internal methods of fetal monitoring are invasive and can increase the risk of infection for the patient and fetus.

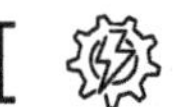

ALERT!

The nurse should advocate for an FSE when the fetus requires continuous monitoring and is difficult to monitor, as long as the cervix allows for insertion and membranes are ruptured.

POP QUIZ 3.2

Given the benefits of EFM using internal methods, why does every pregnant patient not have an internal FSE to measure FHR?

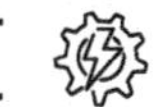

ALERT!

Accelerations that occur while pushing should alert the nurse that this may be the patient's heart rate rather than the FHR. Patient heart rate increases during the pushing stage of labor. The nurse should confirm FHR and patient heart rate to determine that there are two distinct heart rates. A pulse oximeter should be placed on the patient to determine patient heart rate; then an ultrasound should be used to determine FHR. It is important to rule out artifact to ensure that the FHR is accurately measured.

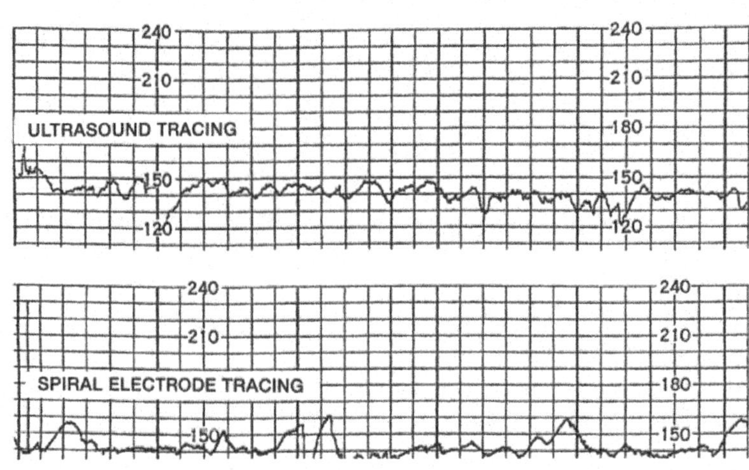

FIGURE 3.2 Accelerations during pushing.

Source: Murray, M., Huelsmann, G., & Koperski, N. (2019). *Essentials of fetal and uterine monitoring.* Springer Publishing Company.

Equipment Failure

- Fetal monitoring equipment can fail to work properly.
- Causes of failure include equipment breaking, power failure, and wrong equipment in use.

Nursing Interventions

- Ensure proper equipment is used.
- Run a sample paper FHR tracing.
- Try a different FHR monitor.
- Try a fetal monitor that is not part of a network.
- Use a handheld Doppler ultrasound transducer and hold it in place continuously if needed.

[] **ALERT!**

Multiple-gestation FHRs may be similar, making it difficult to determine whether there are distinct FHRs. Nurses who cannot determine whether they are seeing the FHRs of separate fetuses should be prepared to call the provider for a bedside ultrasound to determine where each fetus's FHR is located.

UTERINE ACTIVITY ASSESSMENT

Overview

- Uterine activity should be assessed every time the FHR is assessed.
- Adequate contractions are needed for cervical dilation and effacement to occur.
- Uterine contractions are quantified as the number of contractions present in a 10-minute window, averaged over 30 minutes.
- Characteristics of contractions include frequency (how often they occur), duration (how long they last from beginning to end of the contraction), and strength (how strong they are).
- Hormones affect uterine activity: Prior to labor, maternal progesterone levels drop, and estrogen levels rise. The predominance of estrogen increases contractions of the uterus.
- Contractions can be described as normal or abnormal.

Normal Contractions

- Normal: a contraction frequency of one contraction every 2 to 3 minutes (five or fewer contractions in 10 minutes, averaged over a 30-minute window)
- A contraction duration of 60 to 90 seconds
- A contraction strength that is assessed by palpation: Strength is assessed as mild, moderate, or strong. Resting tone (uterine tone between contractions) should be soft (or relaxed).

Abnormal Contractions

- Abnormal: contractions that cannot be characterized as normal frequency, duration, or strength
- Can be characterized as functional dystocia or tachysystole
- Functional dystocia (abnormal, dysfunctional labor): abnormally slow progress of labor and failure of the cervix to dilate; may be due to irregular mild contractions or slow or no change in cervical dilation.
- Tachysystole: more than five contractions in 10 minutes, averaged over a 30-minute window. Can lead to a rising FHR baseline, fewer accelerations, less variability, repetitive decelerations, tachycardia, or bradycardia.

Causes of Abnormal Contractions

- Causes of functional dystocia: labor induction because labor did not start; large fetus; overdistended uterus from polyhydramnios or multiple gestation
- Causes of tachysystole: medications, placental abruption, spontaneous labor, uterotonics (e.g., oxytocin)

Nursing Interventions

- For dysfunctional labor, administer prostaglandins and/or uterotonics as ordered. Amniotomy may be performed.
- For tachysystole: Administer intravenous fluid bolus of lactated Ringer's solution. Decrease rate or discontinue the oxytocin. Remove the dinoprostone insert (medication used to prepare cervix). Withhold the next dose of misoprostol; if no response, terbutaline 0.25 mg subcutaneously may be considered. Reposition patient on the right or left side; administer oxygen, 8 to 10 L per mask.

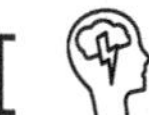

[　　] COMPLICATIONS

Dysfunctional labor can lead to prolonged labor, increasing the risk for chorioamnionitis. Tachysystole can lead to decreased fetal oxygenation, which can lead to fetal hypoxia. In both instances, the risk of Cesarean section is increased.

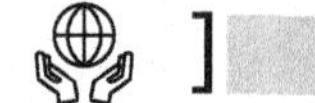

[　　] NURSING PEARL

Resting tone is the pressure exerted by uterine muscle cells when they are at rest between contractions. The strength of resting tone can only be palpated or measured by IUPC. The resting tone should palpate soft or measure 5 to 25 mmHg per IUPC for at least 1 minute to allow the fetus maximum oxygenation between contractions.

[　　] POP QUIZ 3.3

A new nurse is learning about contractions and asks how they would know whether their patient is in tachysystole. How would you educate this nurse?

FETAL ASSESSMENT METHODS

Overview

- Assessments can be used to determine fetal well-being with or without fetal monitoring.
- Assessment methods include auscultation, nonstress test, biophysical profile (BPP), BPP—modified, contraction stress test (CST), fetal movement, umbilical cord blood gas sampling, vibroacoustic stimulation, and fetal scalp stimulation.

Auscultation

Indications

- *Auscultation* is a noninvasive method for low-risk laboring patients that uses the FHR fetoscope, a handheld Doppler ultrasound transducer, or a bedside ultrasound.

Equipment and Procedure

- Fetoscope: A fetoscope is a type of stethoscope used to listen to, or auscultate, the FHR. Place the fetoscope on the patient's abdomen to listen for the fetal heartbeat; count the FHR by using a timer or a watch or clock with a second hand. FHR is calculated in bpm.
- Handheld Doppler ultrasound transducer: A handheld Doppler ultrasound transducer is a small device that is placed on the patient's abdomen and displays the FHR. It requires batteries or a plug to charge it.
- Bedside ultrasound: Bedside ultrasound allows the person using it to hear the FHR and see an ultrasound picture of the fetal heart. Ultrasounds are expensive and may require batteries or a plug to charge them; two-dimensional or three-dimensional ultrasound is available to produce images of the fetus.

Interpretation of Findings

FHR interpretation is discussed in Chapter 4.

Nursing Interventions

- Perform auscultation using available equipment.
- Document FHR assessment.
- Escalate to continuous fetal monitoring if the FHR is not reassuring.
- Check the patient's pulse while checking FHR.

Nonstress Test

Indications

- A nonstress test determines fetal well-being by evaluating fetal oxygenation status and assessing how the FHR responds to fetal movement.
- Antenatal fetal surveillance at 32 0/7 weeks' gestation or later is appropriate for most at-risk or high-risk patients.
- Indications for a nonstress test: advanced patient age, history of complications in previous pregnancy (previous fetal demise, underlying fetal conditions), postterm pregnancy, multiple gestation, placental complications, vaginal bleeding or spotting; gestational hypertension, gestational diabetes mellitus (GDM), cholestasis, preeclampsia (e.g., headache, visual symptoms), Rh sensitization, sickle-cell anemia, substance abuse; decreased fetal movement, fetal tachycardia or bradycardia; intrauterine growth restriction (IUGR); oligohydramnios or polyhydramnios, which may cause IUGR.

Equipment and Procedure

- Position patient in semi-Fowler's or lateral recumbent position.
- Place ultrasound transducer and tocodynamometer on patient's abdomen.
- Use an external fetal monitor to continuously monitor contractions (if any) and FHR.
- To perform vibroacoustic stimulation, have the patient push the button every time fetal movement is felt.
- Monitor the fetus for 20 to 40 minutes.
- Document fetal assessment.

Interpretation of Findings

- Results of the test may show that the fetus is in a sleep cycle.
- Results may indicate the need for further monitoring and testing or for delivery. ▶

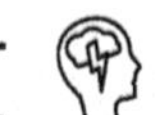

[   ]   COMPLICATIONS

Oligohydramnios (defined as an amniotic fluid volume of 2 cm or less in the single deepest vertical pocket) should prompt further evaluation even if all other components are normal.

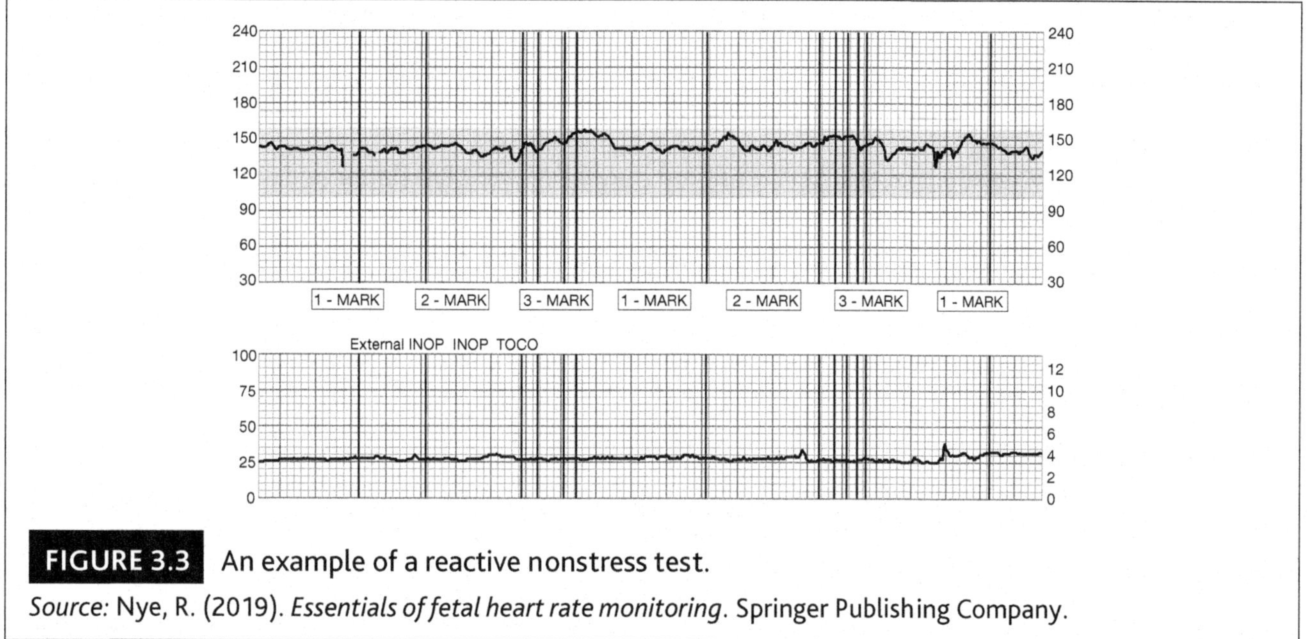

FIGURE 3.3 An example of a reactive nonstress test.

Source: Nye, R. (2019). *Essentials of fetal heart rate monitoring.* Springer Publishing Company.

Interpretation of Findings (continued)

- The findings of a nonstress test are interpreted as either reactive or nonreactive. *Reactive* is considered the normal result (Figure 3.3): For 32 weeks' or greater gestation, two or more accelerations (at least 15 bpm lasting 15 seconds) within a 20-minute period. For less than 32 weeks' gestation, two or more accelerations (at least 10 bpm lasting 10 seconds) within a 20-minute period. Accelerations must be achieved within 40 minutes to be considered reactive. *Nonreactive* findings require further testing, possibly including a BPP (see Figure 3.3).

Nursing Interventions

- Notify provider of results.

Biophysical Profile

Indications

- The BPP consists of a nonstress test based on the FHR monitor and on observations of fetal breathing, movement, tone, and amniotic fluid measurement made by real-time ultrasonography while the patient is lying down.
- The nonstress test may be omitted without compromising test validity if the results of all four ultrasound components of the BPP are within expected ranges.

Equipment and Procedure

- Ultrasound used by the ultrasonographer to determine breathing, movement, tone, and amniotic fluid measurement
- FHR monitor used to assess FHR

Interpretation of Findings

- Expected fetal observations: Fetal breathing—one or more episodes of rhythmic fetal breathing lasting 30 seconds or more within 30 minutes. Fetal movement—three or more discrete body or limb movements within 30 minutes. Fetal tone—one or more episodes of extension of a fetal extremity with return to flexion, or opening or closing of a hand. Amniotic fluid volume—amniotic fluid volume greater than 2 cm in the deepest vertical pocket is considered evidence of adequate amniotic fluid. ▶

[📝]   **POP QUIZ 3.4**

A patient undergoing a nonstress test has been on the monitor for 30 minutes with no accelerations. What could be happening, and what can be done to elicit accelerations?

Interpretation of Findings (continued)
- Results: Each of the five components is assigned a score of either 2 (present) or 0 (not present): Normal composite score: 8 or 10; equivocal composite score: 6; abnormal composite score: 4 or less

Nursing Intervention
- If a BPP presents with abnormal results, the patient may be sent to L&D (labor and delivery) for prolonged fetal monitoring and/or induction of labor.

Biophysical Profile: Modified

Indications
- The modified BPP combines the nonstress test with an amniotic fluid volume assessment performed by ultrasound.

Equipment and Procedure
- FHR monitor used to assess FHR
- Ultrasound used by ultrasonographer or provider to determine amniotic fluid volume

Interpretation of Findings
- Results: Normal—nonstress test is reactive, and the amniotic fluid volume is greater than 2 cm in the deepest vertical pocket. Abnormal—nonstress test is nonreactive, or amniotic fluid volume in the deepest vertical pocket is 2 cm or less.

Nursing Interventions
- If a reactive nonstress test is not achieved within 40 minutes, the patient needs additional fetal monitoring.
- If modified BPP presents abnormal results, the patient may be sent to L&D for prolonged fetal monitoring and/or induction of labor.

Contraction Stress Test

Indications
- The CST is ordered for an atypical nonstress test and/or for concerns about fetal well-being and fetal ability to tolerate labor. Fetal well-being is based on the response of the FHR to uterine contractions. Fetal oxygenation will be transiently worsened by uterine contractions.

Equipment and Procedure
- Procedure: Place patient on FHR monitor. Initiate contractions with nipple stimulation or oxytocin. Assess FHR and contraction pattern with continuous EFM.
- Discontinue nipple stimulation or oxytocin when test is complete.
- If prolonged deceleration or bradycardia of FHR is observed, discontinue test immediately.

 **ALERT!**

A positive CST may indicate the need for a Cesarean section delivery. A patient with abnormal results may be sent to L&D for prolonged fetal monitoring and/or induction of labor.

Interpretation of Findings
- Results are categorized as follows: Negative—no late or significant variable decelerations. Positive—late decelerations after 50% or more of contractions (even if contraction frequency is fewer than three in 10 minutes). Equivocal–suspicious—intermittent late decelerations or significant variable decelerations. Equivocal—decelerations that occur in the presence of contractions more frequently than every 2 minutes or lasting longer than 90 seconds. Unsatisfactory—fewer than three contractions in 10 minutes or an uninterpretable tracing.

Nursing Interventions
- Notify provider of results.

Fetal Movement

Indications

- May be measured by all pregnant patients in the third trimester to assess fetal well-being.

Equipment and Procedure

- Fetal kick count: Fetal kick counts are recommended for all pregnancies after 28 weeks. Instruct patient to move into a side-lying position and to count the number of kicks or fetal movements felt within 2 hours.
- Palpation: The patient can palpate the abdomen to feel fetal movement. The nurse or provider can palpate for fetal movement if the patient is unsure of movement.

Interpretation of Findings

- Ten or more movements within 2 hours is normal.
- Fewer than 10 movements may require further monitoring and/or assessment.

Nursing Interventions

- Educate patient about kick counts.
- Nurse should request a nonstress test for high-risk patients if indicated.
- Results: Document fetal assessment; notify provider of results.

Umbilical Cord Blood Gas Testing

Indications

- Fetal and maternal circulation meets at the placenta, where gas and nutrient exchange occurs.
- The umbilical cord contains three blood vessels: one large umbilical vein (UV) carrying oxygenated blood to the fetus; two small umbilical arteries (UAs) carrying deoxygenated blood that is relatively rich in carbon dioxide and other metabolic waste products from the fetus.
- Oxygen and nutrients diffuse across the placental membrane from maternal arterial blood and are transported to the fetus via the single large UV.
- Fetal blood returns to the placenta following tissue extraction of oxygen and nutrients via the two small UAs.
- The now-deoxygenated blood containing waste products of fetal metabolism (including carbon dioxide) is in maternal circulation and eliminated via maternal lungs and kidneys.
- Sampling umbilical cord gas for an acid–base result provides an objective assessment of fetal metabolic condition at delivery.
- Indications for umbilical cord blood gas testing: Cesarean delivery for fetal compromise; intrapartum fever; Apgar score less than 7 at 5-minute intervals; maternal thyroid disease; multifetal gestation; severe IUGR; placenta abruption; uterine rupture; fetal and maternal blood loss.

Equipment and Procedure

- Clamp and cut a portion of the umbilical cord.
- Obtain a syringe designated for collection of cord blood gas (per facility policy).
- First, collect arterial blood from UA.
- Next, collect blood from UV.

[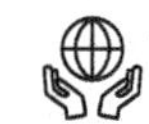]   **NURSING PEARL**

It is important to obtain arterial blood for a cord gas test. When obtaining samples from both types of blood vessels, ensure that one sample is an arterial sample. Arterial cord blood reflects neonatal acid–base status, whereas venous cord blood reflects the combined effect of maternal acid–base status and placental function.

[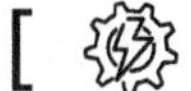]   **ALERT!**

Collect blood from the artery before the vein to prevent collapse of the vessels.

TABLE 3.1 Normal Umbilical Artery and Vein Values

PARAMETER	UMBILICAL ARTERY	UMBILICAL VEIN
pH	7.12–7.35	7.23–7.44
pO_2	6.2–27.6	16.4–40.0
pCO_2	41.9–73.5	28.8–53.3
Bicarbonate	18.8–28.2	17.2–25.6
Base deficit	+9.3 to –1.5	+8.3 to –2.6

Source: Data from Armstrong, L., & Stenson, B. J. (2007). Use of umbilical cord blood gas analysis in the assessment of the newborn. *Archives of Disease in Childhood. Fetal and Neonatal Edition, 92*(6), F430–F434. https://doi.org/10.1136/adc.2006.099846

Interpretation of Findings
- Metabolic acidosis (reduced blood pH and decreased base) implies that sometime during labor, oxygenation of fetal tissues was severely compromised.

Nursing Interventions
- Table 3.1 shows normal UA and UV values. Report abnormal results to provider.

Vibroacoustic Stimulation

Indications
- Vibroacoustic stimulation consists of vibration and sound applied to the patient's abdomen to elicit a fetal response.
- Indications: To awaken the fetus during a nonstress test; to elicit FHR acceleration indicating reactive fetal status.

Equipment and Procedure
- Equipment used is a handheld transducer that delivers an oscillating sound.
- Interpret FHR baseline prior to giving stimulus.
- Perform vibroacoustic stimulation: Maintain continuous FHR tracing; explain the procedure to the patient; position the transducer on the patient's abdomen; apply a stimulus from the transducer for 1 to 2 seconds; assess the FHR tracing after each stimulus to observe for accelerations. If no response, stimulation may be repeated up to three times for progressively longer durations of up to 3 seconds. If still no response, the results are considered nonreactive.
- Continue to maintain continuous FHR tracing after stimulation.

Interpretation of Findings
- See Figure 3.4.

Nursing Interventions
- Avoid performing vibroacoustic stimulation after a deceleration.
- Notify provider if FHR decelerations are noted or if there is no change in FHR tracing.

Fetal Scalp Stimulation

Indications
- Fetal scalp stimulation is used if the fetal scalp is accessible.
- Fetal scalp stimulation is used when no fetal accelerations are detected on the EFM.
- Gentle rubbing of the fetal scalp may elicit an acceleration to rule out metabolic acidosis.

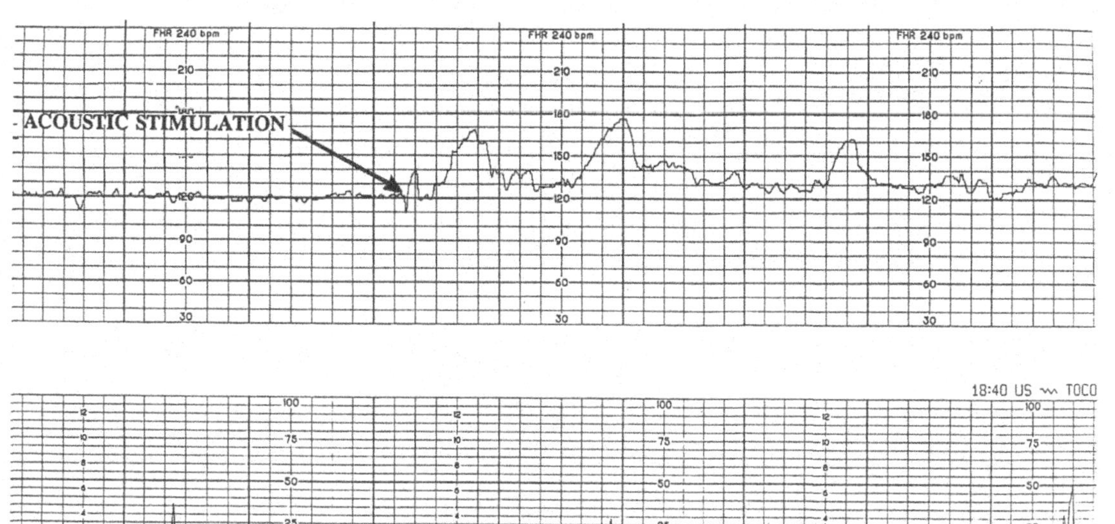

FIGURE 3.4 FHR showing accelerations after vibroacoustic stimulation.

FHR, fetal heart rate.

Source: Murray, M., Huelsmann, G., & Koperski, N. (2019). *Essentials of fetal and uterine monitoring* (5th ed.). Springer Publishing Company.

Equipment and Procedure

- Fetal scalp stimulation may be performed after rupture of membranes if all of the following are true: cervix is dilated at least 3 cm; membranes are ruptured; fetus is engaged at a –1/–2 station.
- Contraindications: cervix closed; infection; amniotic sac intact or not ruptured; fetal distress noted.
- The provider will don a sterile glove and gently touch or rub the fetal scalp for a few seconds to no longer than 15 seconds.

Interpretation of Findings

- An acceleration of the FHR to 15 bpm lasting at least 15 seconds usually reflects a normal fetal scalp pH.
- No acceleration may require interventions based on the FHR.

Nursing Interventions

- Assist the provider at the bedside.
- Assess FHR continuously.
- Assess FHR for accelerations.

[]   **POP QUIZ 3.5**

The nurse has difficulty maintaining the FHR tracing on the monitor while the patient is pushing. The FHR is accelerating with contractions. Is this considered normal? What is the next appropriate step?

RESOURCES

ACOG Committee on Obstetric Practice. (2006). ACOG Committee Opinion No.: Umbilical cord blood gas and acid-base analysis. *Obstetrics & Gynecology*, *108*(5), 1319–1322. https://doi.org/10.1097/00006250-200611000-00058

American College of Obstetricians and Gynecologists. (2009). ACOG Practice Bulletin No. 106: Intrapartum fetal heart rate monitoring: Nomenclature, interpretation, and general management principles. *Obstetrics & Gynecology*, *114*(1), 192–202. https://doi.org/10.1097/aog.0b013e3181aef106

American College of Obstetricians and Gynecologists. (2014a). Obstetric Care Consensus No. 1: Safe prevention of the primary cesarean delivery. *Obstetrics & Gynecology, 123*(3), 693–711. https://doi.org/10.1097/01.aog.0000444441.04111.1d

American College of Obstetricians and Gynecologists. (2014b). Practice Bulletin No. 145: Antepartum fetal surveillance. *Obstetrics & Gynecology, 124*(1), 182–192. https://doi.org/10.1097/01.AOG.0000451759.90082.7b

Armstrong, L., & Stenson, B. J. (2007). Use of umbilical cord blood gas analysis in the assessment of the newborn. *Archives of Disease in Childhood. Fetal and Neonatal Edition, 92*(6), F430–F434. https://doi.org/10.1136/adc.2006.099846

Association of Women's Health, Obstetric and Neonatal Nurses. (2021). *AWHONN position statements.* https://www.awhonn.org/news-advocacy-and-publications/awhonn-position-statements

Basic pattern recognition. (n.d.). Sonic Elephant. http://www.ob-efm.com/efm-basics/basic-pattern-recognition

Groll, C. G. (2016). *Fast facts for the L&D nurse: labor & delivery orientation in a nutshell* (2nd ed.). Springer Publishing Company.

Heelan, L. (2013). Fetal monitoring: creating a culture of safety with informed choice. *Journal of Perinatal Education, 22*(3), 156–165. https://doi.org/10.1891/1058-1243.22.3.156

Kiely, D. J., Oppenheimer, L. W., & Dornan, J. C. (2019). Unrecognized maternal heart rate artefact in cases of perinatal mortality reported to the United States Food and Drug Administration from 2009 to 2019: A critical patient safety issue. *BMC Pregnancy and Childbirth, 19*(1), Article 501. https://doi.org/10.1186/s12884-019-2660-5

Mdoe, P. F., Ersdal, H. L., Mduma, E., Moshiro, R., Kidanto, H., & Mbekenga, C. (2018). Midwives' perceptions on using a fetoscope and Doppler for fetal heart rate assessments during labor: A qualitative study in rural Tanzania. *BMC Pregnancy and Childbirth, 18*, Article 103. https://doi.org/10.1186/s12884-018-1736-y

Murray, M., Huelsmann, G., & Koperski, N. (2019). *Essentials of fetal and uterine monitoring* (5th ed.). Springer Publishing Company.

Nye, R. (2019). *Essentials of fetal heart rate monitoring.* Springer Publishing Company.

Shakouri, F., Iorizzo, L., Edwards, H. M., Vinter, C. A., Kristensen, K., Isberg, P.-E., & Wiberg, N. (2020). Effectiveness of fetal scalp stimulation test in assessing fetal wellbeing during labor, a retrospective cohort study. *BMC Pregnancy and Childbirth, 20*, Article 347. https://doi.org/10.1186/s12884-020-03030-7

4 ELECTRONIC FETAL MONITORING PATTERN RECOGNITION

CATEGORIES OF FETAL HEART RATE TRACINGS

Overview

Three categories of fetal heart rate (FHR) tracings are used to classify the health of the fetus while using electronic fetal monitoring (EFM; Table 4.1).

- Category I: Normal
- Category II: Indeterminate
- Category III: Abnormal

Category I: Normal

- Accelerations present or absent
- Baseline 110 to 160 bpm (see section titled "Fetal Heart Rate Baseline")
- Baseline variability moderate
- Early decelerations present or absent
- Late or variable decelerations absent
- Strongly predictive of normal fetal acid–base status at the time of observation

Nursing Interventions
- No immediate intervention is needed for a normal FHR.
- Continue to observe FHR per facility policy.
- Document findings.

TABLE 4.1 Three Categories of FHR Tracings for Using EFM

CATEGORY I	CATEGORY II	CATEGORY III
All of the following:	*Examples:*	*Either:*
• Baseline 110–160 bpm	• Moderate variability with recurrent late or variable decelerations	• Absent variability with:
• Variability:	• Minimal variability with recurrent variable decelerations	◦ Recurrent late decelerations
◦ Moderate		or
• Late or variable decelerations:	• Absent variability without recurrent decelerations	◦ Recurrent variable decelerations
◦ Absent	• Bradycardia with moderate variability	or
• Early decelerations:	• Prolonged decelerations	◦ Bradycardia
◦ Present or absent		or
• Accelerations:		◦ Sinusoidal pattern
◦ Present or absent		

FHR, fetal heart rate.

Source: Nye, R. (2019). *Essentials of fetal heart rate monitoring.* Springer Publishing Company.

Category II: Indeterminate

- Any tracing not meeting category I or III criteria: absence of induced accelerations after fetal stimulation; absent variability without recurrent decelerations; baseline bradycardia not accompanied by absent baseline variability; baseline tachycardia; marked variability; minimal variability; prolonged deceleration; recurrent late decelerations with moderate variability; recurrent variable decelerations with minimal or moderate variability; variable decelerations

Nursing Interventions
- Interventions depend on the characteristics of FHR variability (or lack of variability) and their cause: Administer intravenous (IV) fluid bolus. Administer oxygen: 8–10 L per nonrebreather mask. Discontinue oxytocin (if running). Notify provider. Reposition patient.
- Monitor FHR closely.

Category III: Abnormal

- Absent variability with any of the following: bradycardia, recurrent late decelerations, recurrent variable decelerations
- Predictive of abnormal fetal acid–base status at the time of observation
- Sinusoidal pattern

Nursing Interventions
- Notify the provider.
- Prepare for urgent delivery.

FETAL HEART RATE BASELINE
Overview

- Baseline must be determined before the FHR can be categorized.
- Baseline is the mean FHR rounded to 5 bpm during a 10-minute segment. The minimum baseline duration must be at least 2 continuous minutes. This segment must exclude accelerations, decelerations, and periods of marked variability.
- Examples of baseline FHR: bradycardia—less than 110 bpm; normal—110 to 160 bpm; tachycardia—more than 160 bpm.
- Measure FHR baseline with properly calibrated EFM equipment (wired or wireless).

Influencing Mechanisms of Fetal Heart Rate Baseline

- Common nonphysiologic mechanisms that influence FHR baseline: fetal—prematurity, sleep cycles; maternal—medications ▶

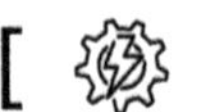

[⚡] ALERT!

There is evidence to suggest that the longer the FHR remains in category II, especially during the last 2 hours before birth, the greater the risk of neonatal morbidity.

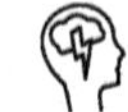

[🧠] COMPLICATIONS

Both bradycardia and tachycardia can indicate fetal complications. Prolonged bradycardia of less than 80 bpm for 3 minutes or longer indicates severe hypoxia of the fetus. Persistent tachycardia of greater than 180 bpm, especially occurring in conjunction with maternal fever, suggests chorioamnionitis.

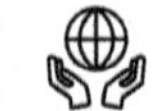

[🌐] NURSING PEARL

If minimum baseline duration is less than 2 minutes, then the baseline is indeterminate. For example, if there are prolonged accelerations or repetitive decelerations that do not allow for any 2 continuous minutes of baseline, then the baseline is indeterminate.

Influencing Mechanisms of Fetal Heart Rate Baseline (*continued*)

- Physiologic mechanisms that influence FHR baseline: fetal—anemia, cardiac arrhythmias, congenital anomalies, preexisting neurologic conditions; maternal—hyperthyroidism, interruption of fetal oxygenation, fever, infection, metabolic acidemia

Nursing Interventions
- Determine and treat abnormal baseline if possible.
- Improve transfer of oxygen to the fetus by increasing placental perfusion: Administer IV fluid; administer supplemental maternal oxygen at 8 to 10 L per nonrebreather mask; change the patient's position; prepare for possible emergent delivery, if indicated.
- Monitor and document: baseline rate and patterns; presence or absence of accelerations and decelerations; interventions and response of the patient and/or fetus; communication with provider.
- Monitor FHR baseline concurrently with uterine contractions and document every 15 to 30 minutes.

FETAL HEART RATE VARIABILITY
Overview

- Classifications (Table 4.2): absent, minimal, moderate, marked
- Variability is fluctuation of the FHR from the baseline in bpm, measured by assessing difference in FHR compared with the baseline of the FHR.
- Variability is the most important determinant of fetal well-being.
- Interventions are based on variability compared to the baseline.
- Interventions may also be influenced by the presence or absence of accelerations and/or decelerations, as well as other factors.

[⚡] **ALERT!**

Manage specific FHR patterns per guidelines. Observe and confirm baseline patterns, document changes or trends over time, and document and evaluate fetal response to possible interruption of oxygen pathways and interventions to improve pathways. An abnormal baseline may be acceptable, such as with a premature fetus or a fetus with a known heart condition; a premature fetus may have an abnormally high baseline. Review the entire FHR tracing, consider maternal and fetal factors that may affect the tracing, and respond appropriately.

[📝] **POP QUIZ 4.1**

The nurse is caring for a pregnant patient, and the fetus has a sudden event of bradycardia of 100 bpm, lasting for 4 minutes. What four steps should the nurse take?

[🧠] **COMPLICATIONS**

A fetus with persistent minimal or absent variability FHR is at risk for severe fetal compromise related to hypoxia.

TABLE 4.2 Classifications of FHR Variability	
CLASSIFICATION	**DEFINITION**
Absent	Undetectable amplitude range
Minimal	Amplitude range of 1–5 bpm
Moderate	Amplitude range of 6–25 bpm
Marked	Amplitude range of greater than 25 bpm

bpm, beats per minute; FHR, fetal heart rate.

Absent and Minimal Variability

- Absent variability has an undetectable amplitude range of the FHR (Figure 4.1).
- Absent variability may be a sign of fetal distress.
- Minimal variability has an amplitude range of 1 to 5 bpm (Figure 4.2).
- Minimal variability may suggest opioid administration to the patient, a fetal sleep cycle, or a premature fetus, or it may be a sign of fetal distress.

Causes

- Fetal arrhythmias and congenital anomalies
- Fetal hypoxemia/acidosis
- Fetal sleep cycles
- Fetal tachycardia
- Maternal medications: anesthetics, barbiturates, narcotics (e.g., para-sympatholytics, anesthetics, or similar), phenothiazines; tranquilizers
- Preexisting fetal neurologic abnormality
- Prematurity

Nursing Interventions

- Notify the provider.
- Discontinue oxytocin if applicable.
- Administer IV fluid bolus.
- Reposition the patient.
- Determine cause.
- Prepare for operative vaginal birth or cesarean section.
- Administer oxygen 8 to 10 L per nonrebreather mask.

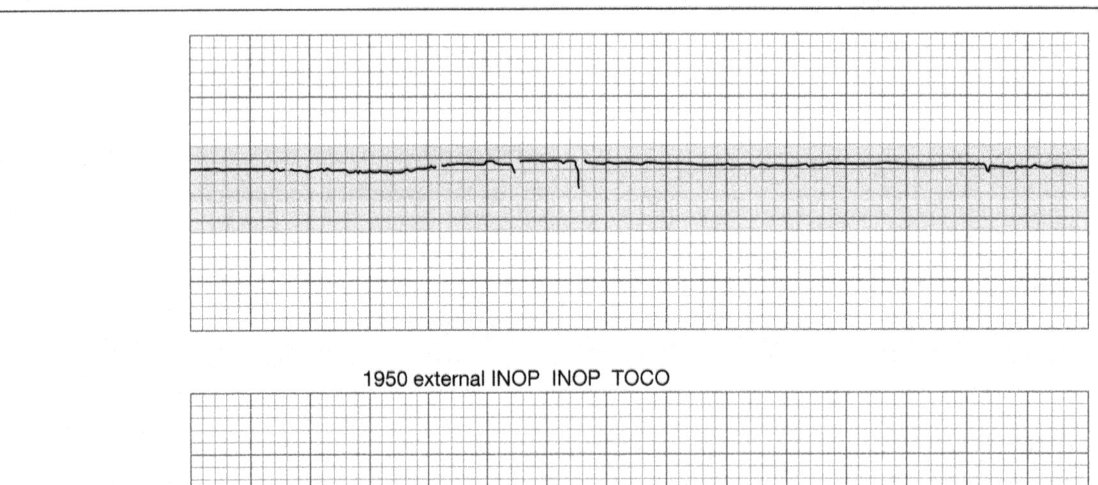

FIGURE 4.1 Absent variability. This tracing shows smooth fetal heartbeat. It is not possible to determine baseline FHR. This is a category II FHR, which requires close monitoring. (Each small square = 10 seconds; each large square = 1 minute.)

FHR, fetal heart rate.

Source: Nye, R. (2019). *Essentials of fetal heart rate monitoring.* Springer Publishing Company.

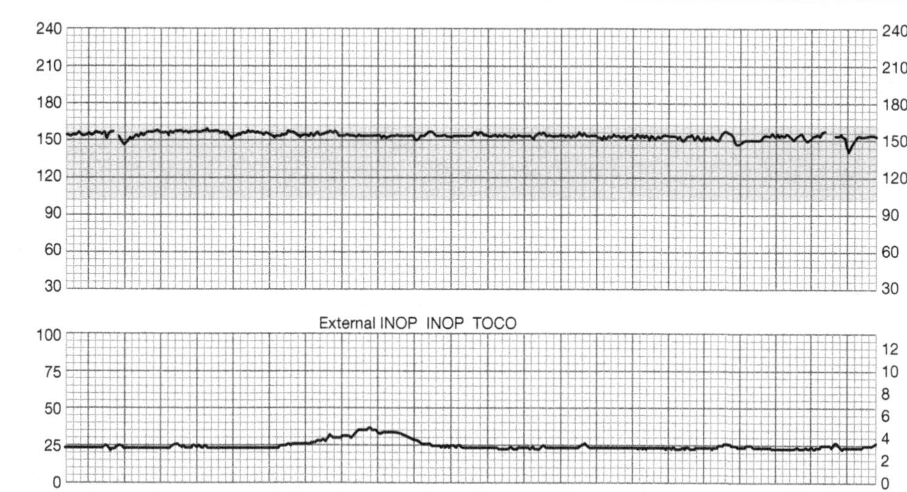

FIGURE 4.2 Minimal variability with a baseline of 150 bpm. This tracing shows some variability (less than 5 bpm) with no accelerations or decelerations. This is a category II FHR and is concerning. It may indicate a fetal sleep cycle or occur after maternal narcotic administration, but if it persists, it requires intervention. (Each small square = 10 seconds; each large square = 1 minute.)

bpm, beats per minute; FHR, fetal heart rate.

Source: Nye, R. (2019). *Essentials of fetal heart rate monitoring* (Fig. 3.6). Springer Publishing Company.

Nursing Interventions (continued)
- Document all interventions performed.
- Monitor FHR.
- Evaluate fetal response to interventions.

Moderate Variability

- Has an amplitude range of 6 to 25 bpm
- Signifies the absence of fetal acidosis (Figure 4.3)
- Is reflective of normal variability for a well-oxygenated fetus

Causes
- Nonacidotic fetus (normal)

Nursing Interventions
- Document FHR interpretation per facility policy.
- Monitor FHR per facility policy, as no immediate interventions are needed.

Marked Variability

- Has an amplitude range of greater than 25 bpm (Figure 4.4)
- Is not related to neonatal morbidity, although it has been correlated with abnormal arterial cord blood gases

Causes
- Fetal stimulation: contractions, vaginal examination
- Maternal medications: albuterol, terbutaline
- Maternal substances: cocaine, methamphetamine, nicotine
- Mild hypoxemia

[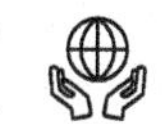]   **NURSING PEARL**

Moderate variability reliably predicts the absence of fetal metabolic acidosis at the time it is observed.

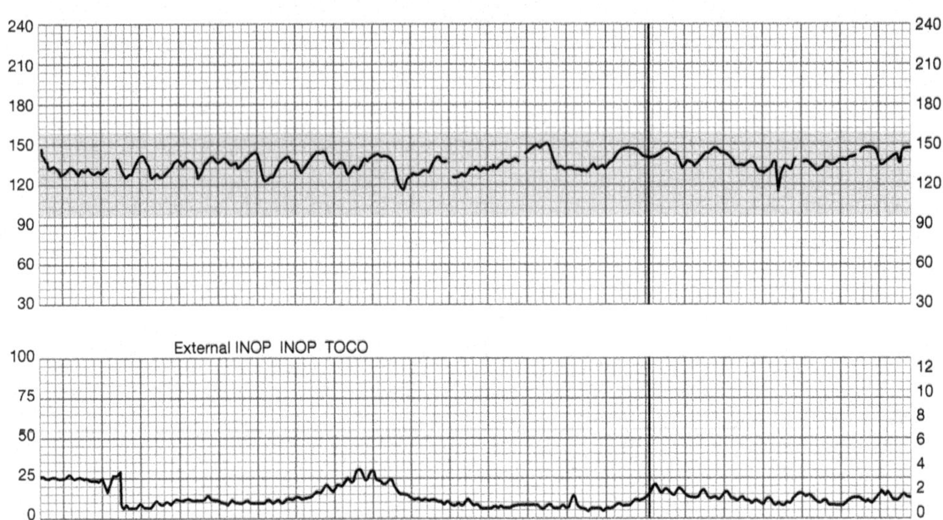

FIGURE 4.3 Moderate variability with a baseline of 135 bpm. There are accelerations with a peak of 15 bpm, lasting 15 seconds or more. There are no decelerations. (Each small square = 10 seconds; each large square = 1 minute.) This is a normal, category I FHR that demonstrates a nonacidotic fetus. This FHR does not require any intervention other than observation and documentation of findings.

bpm, beats per minute; FHR, fetal heart rate.

Source: Nye, R. (2019). *Essentials of fetal heart rate monitoring.* Springer Publishing Company.

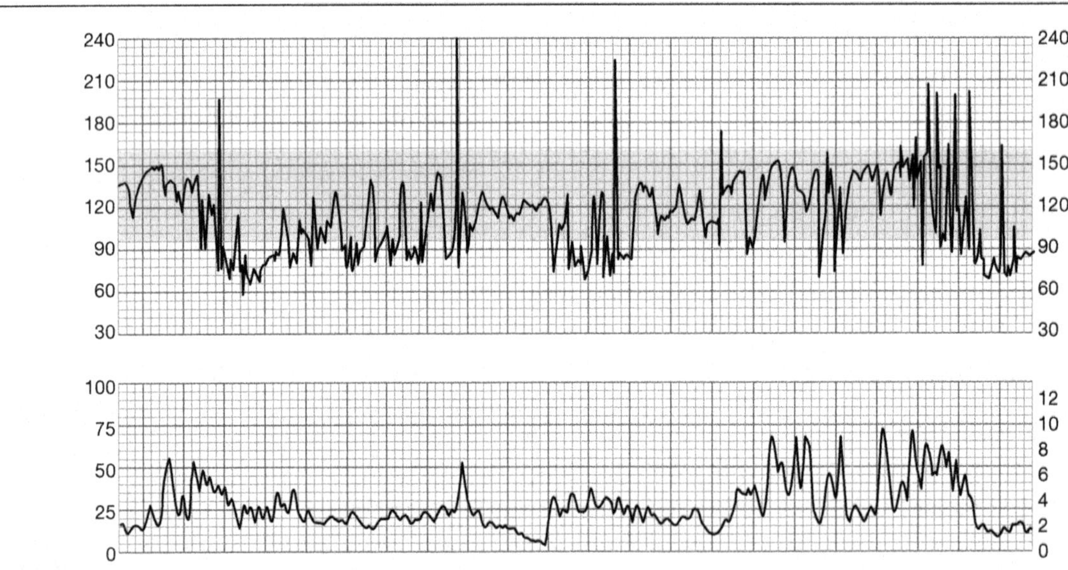

FIGURE 4.4 Marked variability. The FHR is greater than 25 bpm, making it impossible to determine the baseline or determine accelerations or decelerations. (Each small square = 10 seconds; each large square = 1 minute.) This is a category II FHR that needs further monitoring and notification of provider.

bpm, beats per minute; FHR, fetal heart rate.

Source: Nye, R. (2019). *Essentials of fetal heart rate monitoring.* Springer Publishing Company.

Nursing Interventions

In order of priority:

- Notify the provider.
- Monitor the patient closely.
- Apply a fetal scalp electrode for more accurate reading of FHR variability.
- Determine the cause.
- Document all interventions performed.
- Monitor FHR.
- Evaluate fetal response to interventions.

FETAL HEART RATE ACCELERATIONS

Overview

- Adequate accelerations are as follows: less than 32 weeks' gestation—greater than or equal to 10 bpm above baseline for at least 10 seconds; greater than 32 weeks' gestation—greater than or equal to 15 bpm above baseline for at least 15 seconds
- An *FHR acceleration* is an abrupt increase from FHR baseline with time of onset to peak of acceleration less than 30 seconds, lasting less than 2 minutes (Figure 4.5).
- A *prolonged acceleration* is an increase in heart rate that lasts longer than 2 minutes but less than 10 minutes.

[]   **POP QUIZ 4.2**

What is the most important characteristic of FHR tracings in determining fetal well-being?

[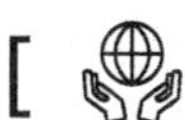]   **NURSING PEARL**

Any acceleration or deceleration that lasts longer than 10 minutes is considered a change in FHR baseline.

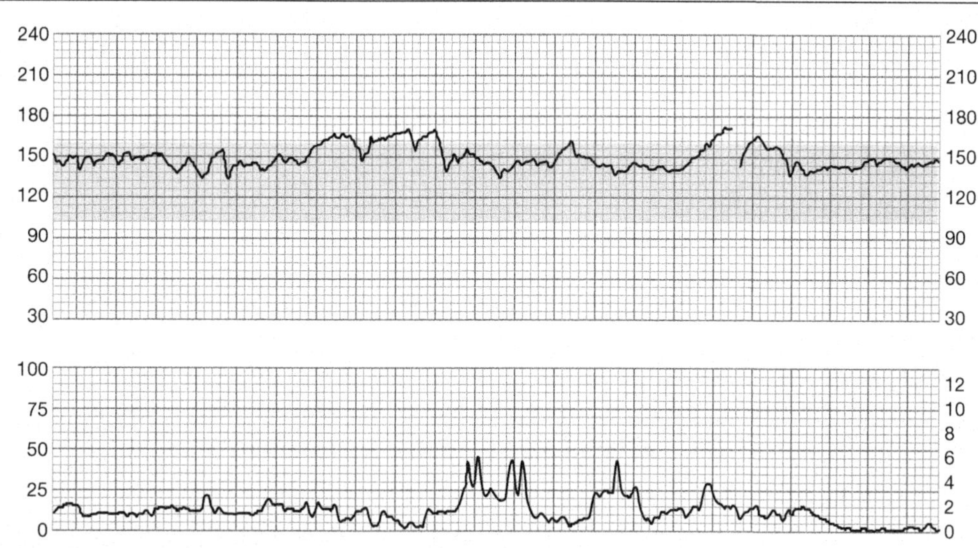

FIGURE 4.5 FHR showing accelerations. The FHR baseline is 145 bpm with moderate variability. There are accelerations that are at least 15 bpm above baseline and last for at least 15 seconds. There are no decelerations. (Each small square = 10 seconds; each large square = 1 minute.) This is a category I FHR.

bpm, beats per minute; FHR, fetal heart rate.

Source: Nye, R. (2019). *Essentials of fetal heart rate monitoring.* Springer Publishing Company.

Causes

There are many possible causes of FHR acceleration, which may include:

- Fetal movement
- Vaginal examinations
- Uterine contractions
- Umbilical vein compression
- Fetal scalp stimulation
- External acoustic stimulation

Nursing Interventions

- This is a normal, reactive pattern.
- Monitor FHR per facility policy, as no immediate interventions are needed.

FETAL HEART RATE DECELERATIONS

Overview

- Decelerations are a decrease of FHR below baseline. They are considered *intermittent* if they occur with less than 50% of contractions in a 20-minute period; they are considered *recurrent* if they occur with more than 50% of contractions in a 20-minute period
- Types of decelerations: early decelerations, late decelerations, periodic or episodic decelerations, prolonged decelerations, variable decelerations

[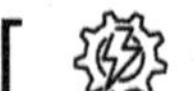]   **ALERT!**

Early decelerations are not usually seen in early labor. If they are observed in early labor, it could be due to breech presentation. Verify fetal position by vaginal examination or ultrasound.

Early Decelerations

- Are gradual decreases in FHR and may be observed as labor progresses.
- Measure more than 30 seconds from onset of deceleration to nadir (the lowest point of a deceleration; occurs with the peak of a contraction; Figure 4.6).
- May be observed as labor progresses.
- Are not associated with adverse outcomes.

Causes

- Breech presentation
- Fetal head compression (Figure 4.7)
- Thought to represent a fetal autonomic response to changes in intracranial pressure and/or cerebral blood flow caused by compression of the fetal head during uterine contractions

Nursing Interventions

- Monitor FHR per facility policy, as no immediate interventions are needed. These are normal decelerations.

Late Decelerations

- Late decelerations are a gradual decrease in FHR with onset of deceleration to nadir greater than 30 seconds (Figure 4.8).
- Onset of the deceleration occurs after the beginning of the contraction, and the nadir of the contraction occurs after the peak of the contraction. ▶

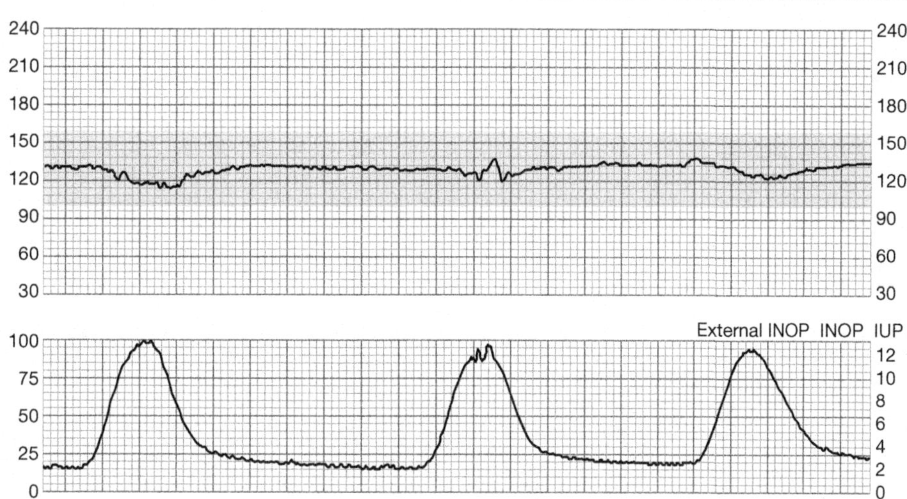

FIGURE 4.6 Early decelerations observed, mirroring contractions. The FHR baseline is 130 bpm, with minimal variability. There are no accelerations or decelerations. (Each small square = 10 seconds; each large square = 1 minute.) The tracing is category II because of the variability. The decelerations are a normal finding.

bpm, beats per minute; FHR, fetal heart rate.

Source: Nye, R. (2019). *Essentials of fetal heart rate monitoring.* Springer Publishing Company.

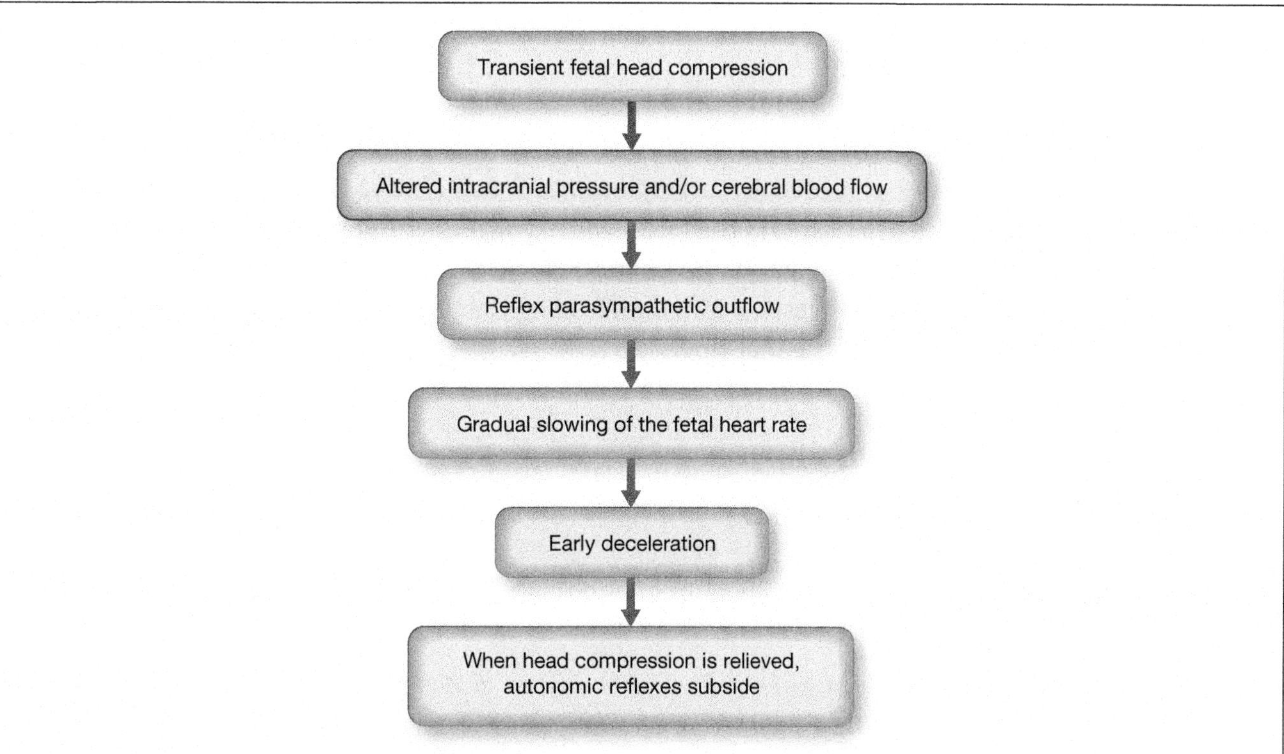

FIGURE 4.7 Pathophysiology of early deceleration. Fetal head compression triggers blood flow, which triggers the parasympathetic reflex, slowing the FHR.

FHR, fetal heart rate.

Source: Nye, R. (2019). *Essentials of fetal heart rate monitoring.* Springer Publishing Company.

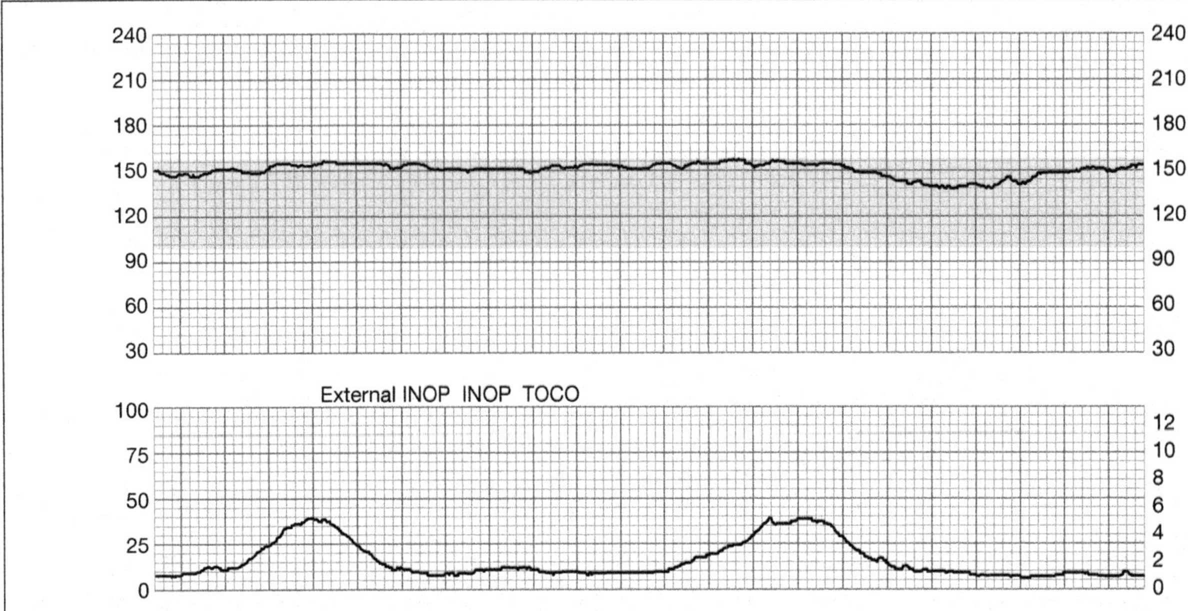

FIGURE 4.8   Late decelerations. The deceleration begins with the contraction and ends after the contraction finishes, making it a late deceleration. The FHR baseline is 150 bpm with minimal variability. (Each small square = 10 seconds; each large square = 1 minute.) This is a category II FHR, which requires interventions.

bpm, beats per minute; FHR, fetal heart rate.

Source: Nye, R. (2019). *Essentials of fetal heart rate monitoring.* Springer Publishing Company.

Late Decelerations (*continued*)

- Late deceleration is usually preceded by uteroplacental insufficiency. Decreased oxygen from the placenta to the fetus causes hypoxemia in the fetus, which triggers a response from the chemoreceptors to the baroreceptors, leading to a parasympathetic response and a late deceleration (Figure 4.9). Decreased oxygen levels can cause vasoconstriction, leading to hypertension; hypertension stimulates a baroreceptor-mediated vagal response that slows the FHR.

Causes
- Diabetes
- Excessive uterine contractions
- Fetal intrauterine growth restriction (IUGR)
- Hypertensive disorders
- Maternal hypotension
- Maternal hypoxemia
- Placental abruption

Nursing Interventions
- Administer IV hydration.
- Administer oxygen.
- Correct any hypotension with IV fluid bolus, medications, and/or blood products.
- Discontinue oxytocin.
- Place patient in the lateral position.
- Notify provider if late deceleration persists.

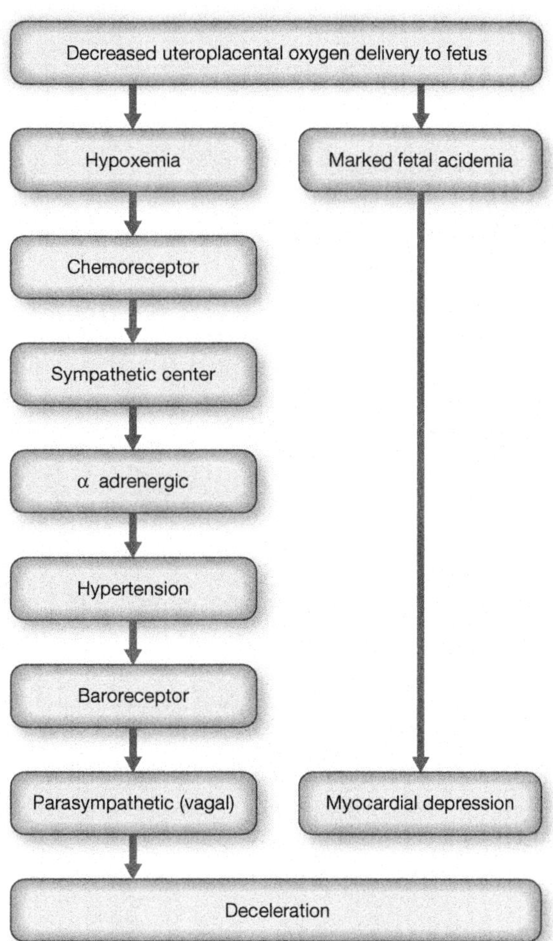

FIGURE 4.9 Pathophysiology of a late deceleration. Decreased oxygen from the placenta to the fetus causes hypoxemia, which triggers a response from the chemoreceptors to the baroreceptors, leading to a parasympathetic response and a late deceleration. If the placenta does not deliver oxygen to the fetus for a prolonged period, acidemia can occur, leading to myocardial depression and late decelerations.

bpm, beats per minute; FHR, fetal heart rate.

Source: Nye, R. (2019). *Essentials of fetal heart rate monitoring.* Springer Publishing Company.

Variable Decelerations

- *Variable deceleration* is a visually apparent, abrupt decrease in FHR. Onset of deceleration to nadir is less than 30 seconds. Heart rate is at least 15 bpm below baseline, lasting between 15 seconds and 2 minutes (Figure 4.10).
- Pathophysiology of variable decelerations (Figure 4.11): Variable decelerations are vagally mediated through chemoreceptors or baroreceptors. Decreased venous return causes a baroreceptor-mediated acceleration and decreased arterial oxygen tension secondary to complete cord compression. In a premature fetus, variable decelerations can occur with head compression secondary to vagal nerve activation from fetal movement.

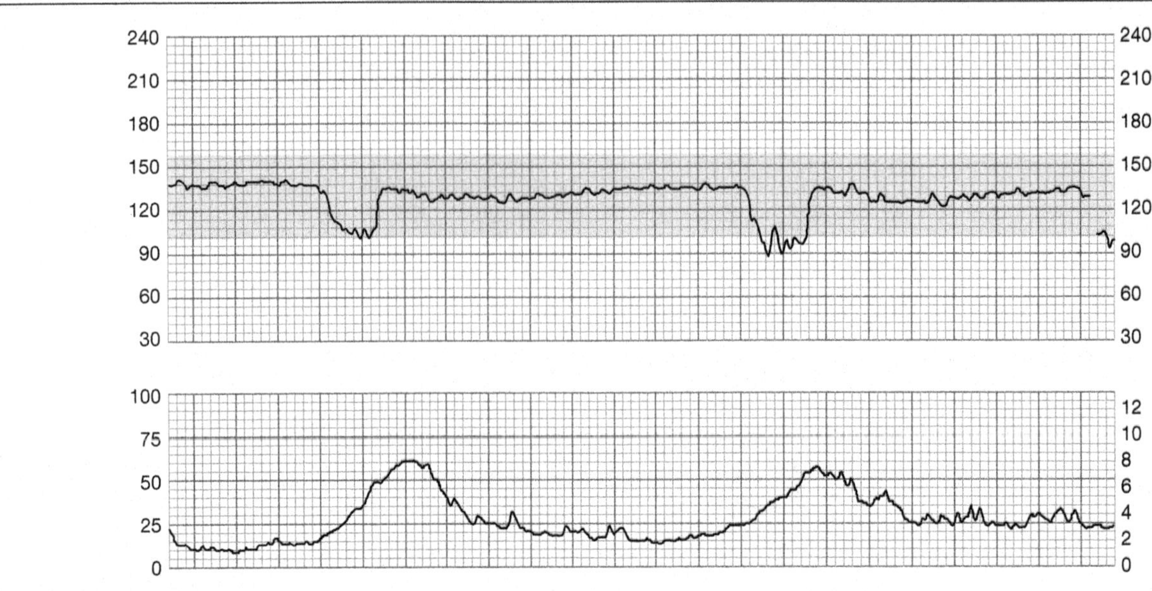

FIGURE 4.10   Variable decelerations observed. The baseline is 135 bpm. The FHR shows moderate variability with no accelerations and variable decelerations. (Each small square = 10 seconds; each large square = 1 minute.) This is a category II FHR.

bpm, beats per minute; FHR, fetal heart rate.

Source: Nye, R. (2019). *Essentials of fetal heart rate monitoring.* Springer Publishing Company.

Causes

- Umbilical cord compression, which can be caused by the cord wrapping around the fetus's body or neck (also called *nuchal cord*)
- Fetal pressure on umbilical cord
- Prolapsed umbilical cord

Nursing Interventions

- Administer oxygen.
- Change position of patient to rest where FHR pattern is most improved. The Trendelenburg position (supine with feet higher than head) may be helpful.
- Assess for umbilical cord prolapse or imminent delivery with vaginal examination. Umbilical cord prolapse requires emergent cesarean section.
- Prepare for amnioinfusion.
- Discontinue oxytocin.
- Modify patient's pushing to every second or third contraction.

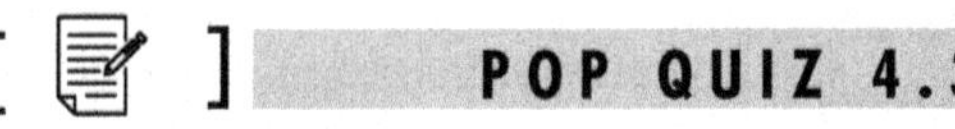

POP QUIZ 4.3

Which type of deceleration would most likely be alleviated with amnioinfusion?

Periodic or Episodic Decelerations

- *Episodic patterns* are those not associated with uterine contractions.
- *Periodic patterns* are those associated with uterine contractions.
- Early and late decelerations are periodic.
- Variable decelerations can be periodic or episodic.

Causes

Cause depends on the type of deceleration: early, late, or variable.

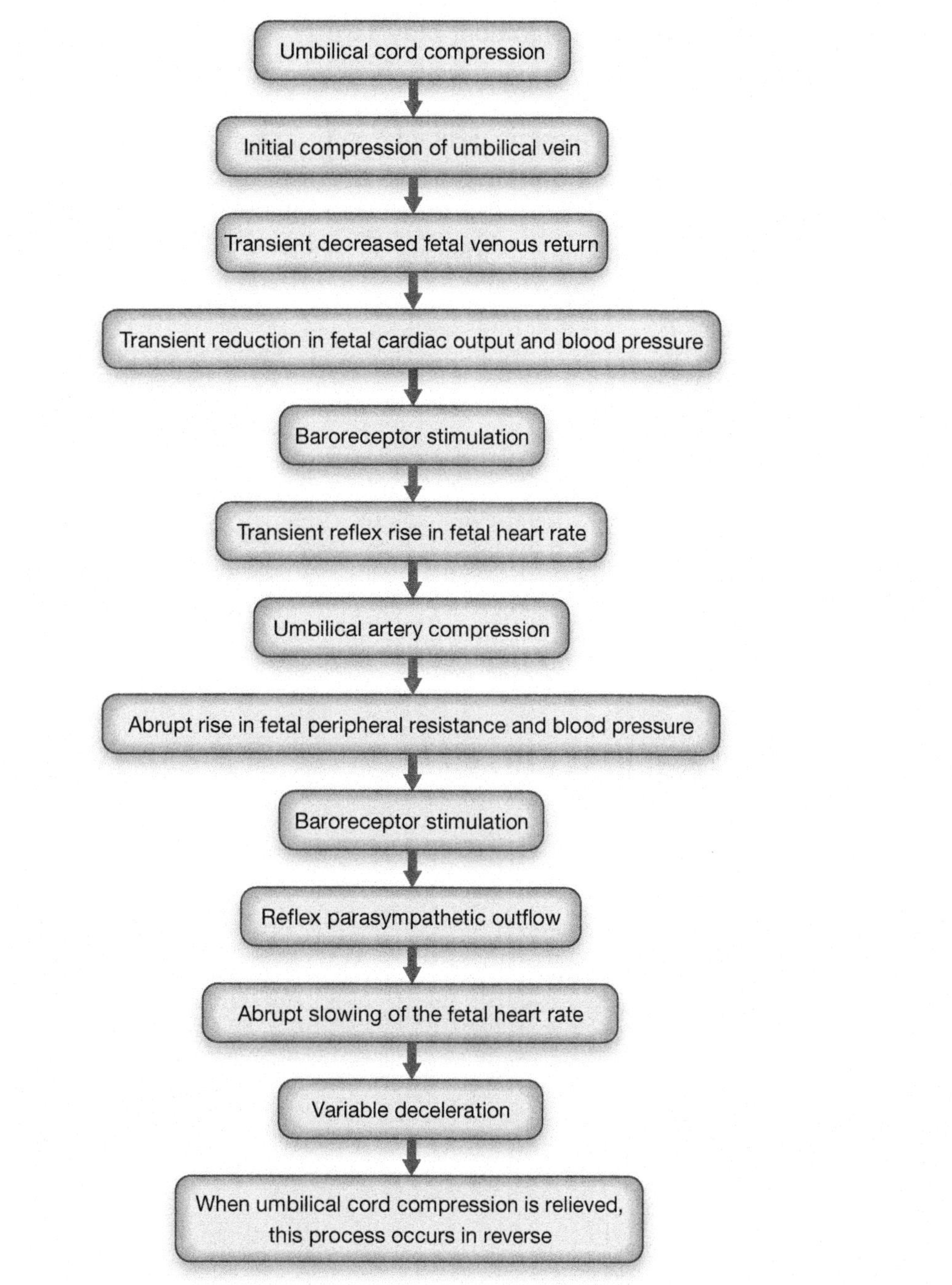

FIGURE 4.11 Pathophysiology of a variable deceleration. Umbilical cord compression compresses the umbilical vein, leading to decreased venous return, which can trigger baroreceptor stimulation and a transient rise in the FHR. This can be seen as a rise in baseline right before the deceleration, which occurs when the artery is compressed, causing a rise in peripheral resistance. This then causes baroreceptor stimulation, which leads to parasympathetic reflux and an abrupt slowing of the FHR.

FHR, fetal heart rate.

Source: Nye, R. (2019). *Essentials of fetal heart rate monitoring.* Springer Publishing Company.

Nursing Interventions
Intervention depends on the type of deceleration: early, late, or variable.

Prolonged Decelerations

- A *prolonged deceleration* is a decrease in FHR of greater than 15 bpm, measured from the most recently determined baseline rate.
- A prolonged deceleration lasts at least 2 minutes but less than 10 minutes (Figure 4.12).

Causes
- Artifact
- Umbilical cord compression
- Umbilical cord prolapse
- Maternal hypotension
- Maternal seizure
- Placental abruption
- Uterine hyperactivity
- Uterine rupture

[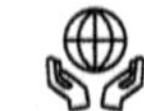]   **NURSING PEARL**

VEAL CHOP is a mnemonic used to help remember FHR patterns (VEAL) and their causes (CHOP):
- Heart rate pattern
  - Variable decelerations
  - Early decelerations
  - Accelerations
  - Late decelerations
- Cause
  - Cord compression
  - Head compression
  - Okay
  - Placental insufficiency

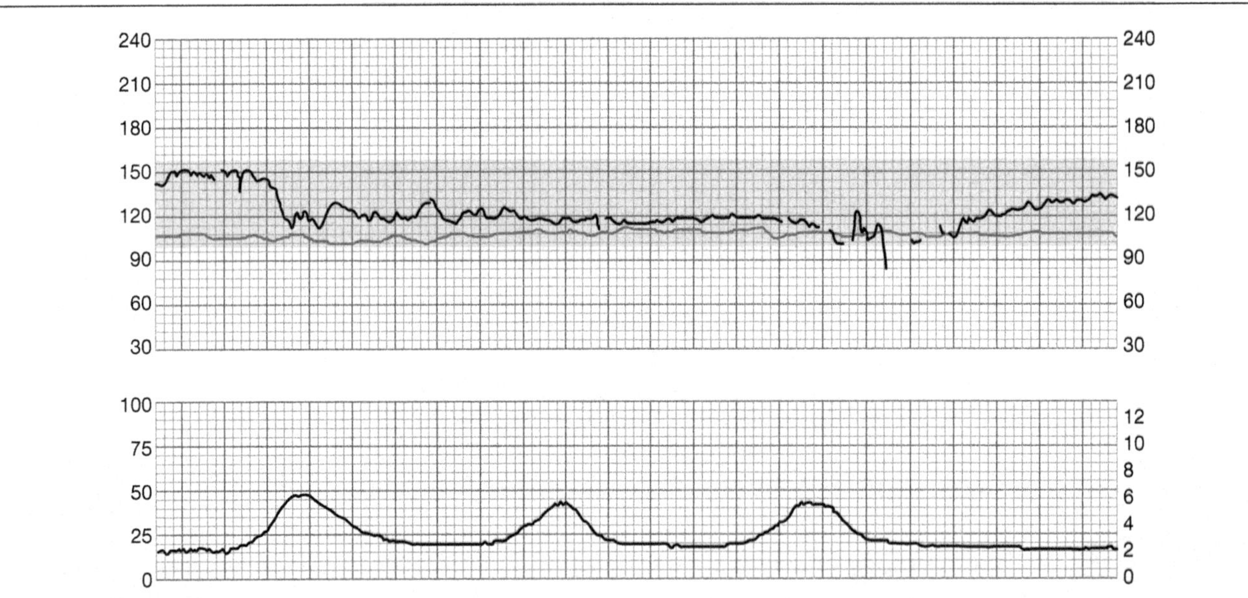

FIGURE 4.12   A prolonged deceleration lasting approximately 6 minutes. The baseline cannot be determined because 2 minutes of baseline are not shown here. There is minimal to moderate variability and no accelerations. (Each small square = 10 seconds; each large square = 1 minute.) This is a category II FHR that requires interventions.

FHR, fetal heart rate.

Source: Nye, R. (2019). *Essentials of fetal heart rate monitoring.* Springer Publishing Company.

Nursing Interventions
- Administer IV hydration.
- Administer oxygen.
- Correct any hypotension with IV fluid bolus of normal saline or lactated Ringer's solution, medication, and/or blood products.
- Discontinue oxytocin.
- Place patient in the lateral position.

FETAL ARRYTHMIAS

Overview

- Arrhythmias are classified as bradycardia, tachycardia, pseudo-sinusoidal, and sinusoidal.
- *Fetal arrhythmias* are abnormalities in the FHR baseline that last longer than 10 minutes.
- If an arrhythmia is observed during intermittent fetal monitoring, the patient should be placed on continuous monitoring, and the nurse should assess every 15 minutes or per institutional policy.

Bradycardia

- *Bradycardia* refers to FHR less than 110 bpm in a term fetus or less than 120 bpm in a preterm fetus, lasting longer than 10 minutes.
- Some fetuses have a naturally low baseline FHR, but low-baseline FHR can indicate complications in other cases (Figure 4.13).

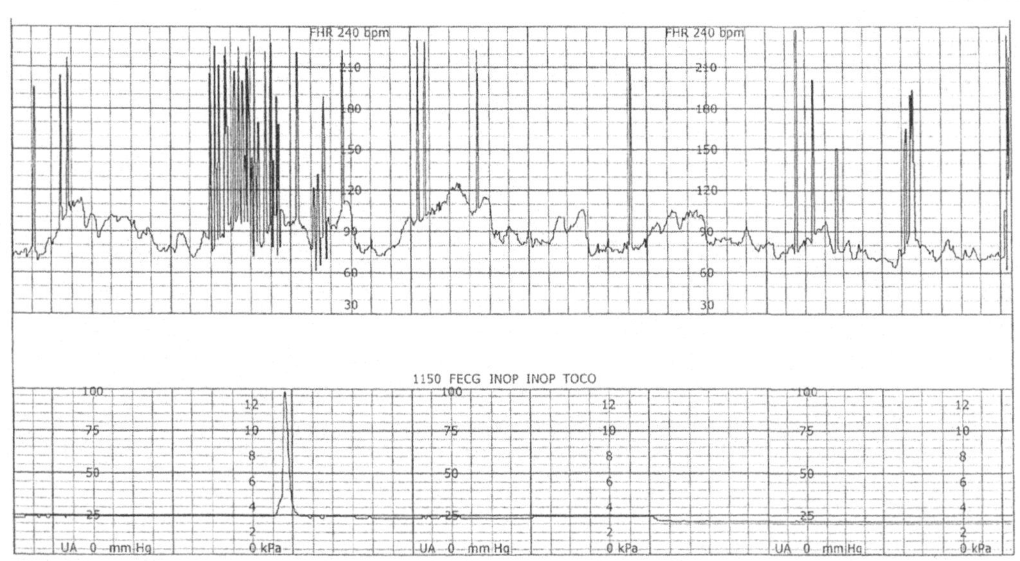

FIGURE 4.13 FHR showing bradycardia with a baseline FHR of approximately 85 bpm to 90 bpm. (Each small square = 10 seconds; each large square = 1 minute). There is moderate variability and accelerations. This is a category III FHR that requires immediate attention.

bpm, beats per minute; FHR, fetal heart rate.

Source: Murray, M., Huelsmann, G., and Koperski, N. (2019). *Essentials of fetal and uterine monitoring* (5th ed.). Springer Publishing Company.

Causes

- Asphyxia
- Fetal heart block
- Hypoxia with or without metabolic acidosis
- Maternal hypotension (e.g., after epidural placement)
- Metabolic acidosis
- Placental abruption
- Rapid fetal descent
- Tachysystole
- Umbilical cord prolapse
- Uterine rupture

Nursing Interventions

- Increase fetal perfusion and oxygenation: Administer oxygen; discontinue oxytocin; start IV hydration (normal saline or lactated Ringer's solution).
- Notify provider of new-onset bradycardia. Prepare for an emergency cesarean section if vaginal delivery is not expected in the next few minutes.
- Place patient in lateral position.

[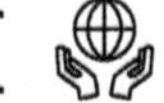]   **COMPLICATIONS**

Tachycardia without accelerations but with decreased baseline variability has been demonstrated to cause fetal hypoxia, hypercarbia, and metabolic acidosis.

Tachycardia

- *Tachycardia* is defined as FHR greater than 160 bpm lasting longer than 10 minutes (Figure 4.14). Tachycardia can be related to vagal suppression and/or sympathetic dominance.

Causes

- Chorioamnionitis
- Fetal anemia
- Fetal hypoxia
- Fetal tachyarrhythmia
- Fetal heart failure
- Maternal fever
- Medications: beta sympathomimetics, hydroxyzine pamoate, phenothiazines, tocolytic (e.g., terbutaline)

Nursing Interventions

- Assess patient to evaluate and treat cause of fetal tachycardia.
- Notify provider.
- Treat patient fever and infection per provider orders.

[☠]   **NURSING PEARL**

Maternal fever is the most common cause of new-onset fetal tachycardia.

Pseudo-Sinusoidal

- *Pseudo-sinusoidal* rhythm is a smooth, wave-like, undulating pattern with a cycle frequency of 3 to 5 minutes.
- It is characterized by fluctuations in the baseline that are regular in amplitude and frequency.
- Pattern stops after 30 to 40 minutes.

Causes

- Fetal sleep cycle
- Maternal narcotics

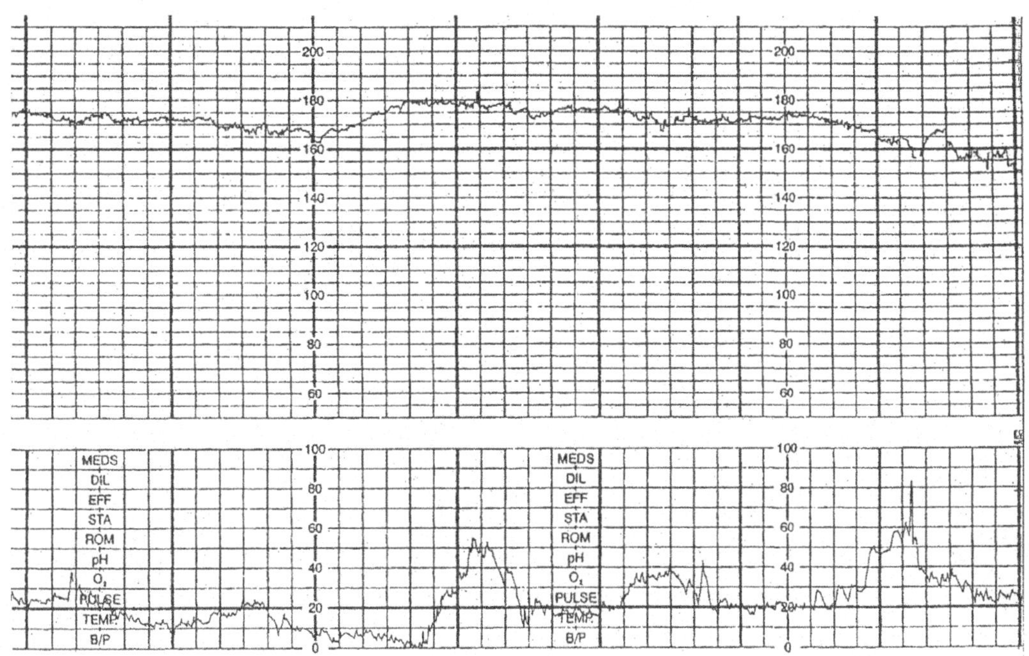

FIGURE 4.14   FHR showing tachycardia with a baseline FHR of approximately 170 bpm. The variability is moderate, with accelerations and no decelerations, although the end of the tracing may be the beginning of a deceleration. (Each small square = 10 seconds; each large square = 1 minute.) This is a category II FHR tracing, which requires interventions.

bpm, beats per minute; FHR, fetal heart rate.

Source: Murray, M., Huelsmann, G., & Koperski, N. (2019). *Essentials of fetal and uterine monitoring* (5th ed.). Springer Publishing Company.

Nursing Interventions
- Monitor for at least 20 minutes if the patient received narcotics or to determine whether the cause of pattern is a fetal sleep cycle.
- Notify the provider if pattern persists.

Sinusoidal

- *Sinusoidal* rhythm is a smooth, wave-like, undulating pattern with a cycle frequency of 3 to 5 minutes persisting for at least 20 minutes (Figure 4.15).
- It is characterized by fluctuations in the baseline, which are regular in amplitude and frequency.
- A sinusoidal pattern is an ominous FHR pattern associated with neonatal morbidity and mortality.

Causes
- Fetal hypoxia
- Severe fetal anemia, such as abruption or ABO incompatibility

Nursing Interventions
- Prepare for emergent delivery, to include cesarean section if vaginal delivery is not imminent.

[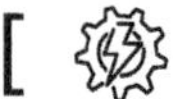]   **ALERT!**

It is important for the nurse to determine the cause for a pseudo-sinusoidal pattern by looking at the overall tracing for longer than 20 minutes. Narcotic administration and fetal sleep cycles can cause a pseudo-sinusoidal pattern. Consider risk factors for a sinusoidal pattern, and if the nurse is unsure of the cause, notify the provider.

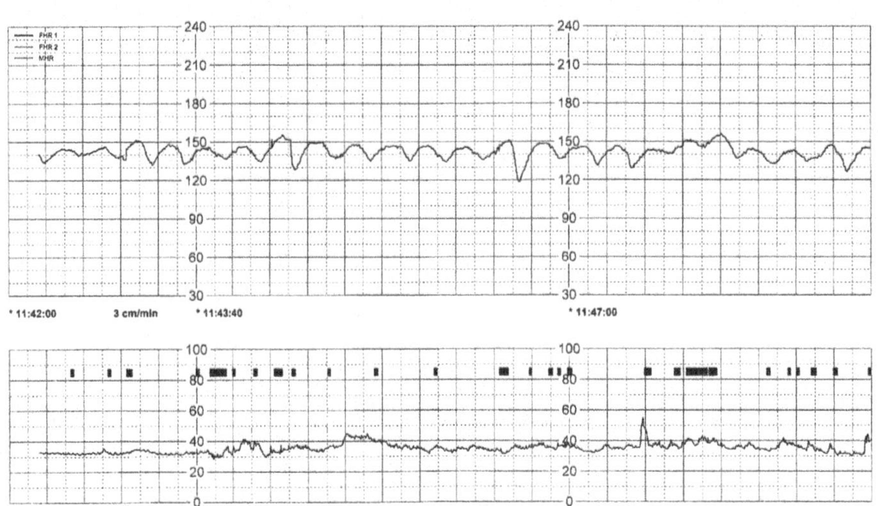

FIGURE 4.15 A sinusoidal pattern. (Each small square = 10 seconds; each large square = 1 minute.) The baseline of this FHR is approximately 140 bpm. The variability is not determined in a sinusoidal pattern. There are no accelerations or decelerations. This is a category III FHR, which requires immediate interventions.

bpm, beats per minute; FHR, fetal heart rate.

Source: Murray, M., Huelsmann, G., & Koperski, N. (2019). *Essentials of fetal and uterine monitoring* (5th ed.). Springer Publishing Company.

RESOURCES

American College of Obstetricians and Gynecologists. (2010). Practice Bulletin No. 116: Management of intrapartum fetal heart rate tracings. *Obstetrics & Gynecology, 116*(5), 1232–1240. https://doi.org/10.1097/AOG.0b013e3182004fa9

Association of Women's Health, Obstetric and Neonatal Nurses. (2015). *Fetal heart monitoring: Principles and practices* (5th ed.). Kendall Hunt.

Cahill, A. G., & Spain, J. (2015). Intrapartum fetal monitoring. *Clinical Obstetrics and Gynecology, 58*(2), 263–268. https://doi.org/10.1097/GRF.0000000000000109

Miller, L. A., Miller, D. A., & Cypher, R. L. (2017). *Mosby's pocket guide to fetal monitoring: a multidisciplinary approach.* Elsevier.

Murray, M., Huelsmann, G., & Koperski, N. (2019). *Essentials of fetal and uterine monitoring* (5th ed.). Springer Publishing Company.

National Certification Corporation. (2016). *2016 NCC monograph free version.pdf.* https://ncc-efm.org/filz/2016%20NCC%20Monograph%20Free%20Version.pdf

Nye, R. (2019). *Essentials of fetal heart rate monitoring.* Springer Publishing Company.

Polnaszek, B., López, J. D., Clark, R., Raghuraman, N., Macones, G. A., & Cahill, A. G. (2020). Marked variability in intrapartum electronic fetal heart rate patterns: Association with neonatal morbidity and abnormal arterial cord gas. *Journal of Perinatology, 40*(1), 56–62. https://doi.org/10.1038/s41372-019-0520-9

Sweha, A., Hacker, T. W., & Nuovo, J. (1999). Interpretation of the electronic fetal heart rate during labor. *American Family Physician, 59*(9), 2487–2500. https://www.aafp.org/pubs/afp/issues/1999/0501/p2487.html

5 COMPLICATIONS

FETAL COMPLICATIONS

- In this chapter, fetal complications are partially organized using the categories from Table 2.1 (see Chapter 2): environmental conditions, maternal respiratory system, maternal blood flow, maternal seizure, uterus; placenta, umbilical cord, fetus, other maternal complications, complications of labor.

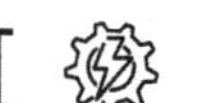

[**ALERT!**]

All fetal complications can lead to fetal demise if not treated immediately.

ENVIRONMENTAL CONDITIONS

- Pollution
- Smoke (can include particulate matter from fires, air pollution, and secondhand smoke from tobacco products)

Nursing Interventions

- Assess patient via continuous electronic fetal monitoring (EFM) to observe and identify fetal response to any disruption of the maternal–fetal oxygen pathway.
- Implement nursing interventions to increase blood flow to improve uteroplacental circulation and promote fetal oxygenation: Reposition patient to a lateral position. Administer intravenous (IV) fluid bolus. Administer supplemental oxygen. Modify pushing efforts. Decrease oxytocin rate by decreasing oxytocin, removing prostaglandin E2 insert, and/or withholding next dose of misoprostol.

MATERNAL RESPIRATORY SYSTEM

MATERNAL LUNGS

- Respiratory depression affects the maternal lungs in the maternal–fetal oxygen pathway.
- *Respiratory depression* is defined as slow and ineffective breathing.
- Symptoms of respiratory depression include feeling tired and short of breath.
- Causes of respiratory depression include: chronic lung diseases such as asthma and cystic fibrosis, hypoventilation, neuromuscular disease, and obstructive sleep apnea.
- Abnormal maternal respiratory findings can affect fetal oxygenation because they can cause impaired gas exchange.

Nursing Interventions

- Maintain continuous fetal heart rate (FHR) tracing.
- Determine cause of respiratory depression and treat underlying cause.
- Monitor pulse oximetry, respiratory rate, and respiratory status.
- Auscultate breath sounds to determine whether lungs are clear bilaterally.
- Administer supplemental oxygen.
- Administer medication as ordered to improve lung function and gas exchange.

MATERNAL BLOOD FLOW

MATERNAL CARDIAC DISEASE AND BLOOD DISORDERS

- Blood disorders include anemia, sickle cell anemia, and thalassemia.
- Cardiac disease includes congestive heart failure, cardiomyopathy, heart rhythm disorders, heart valve disorders, and congenital heart disease.
- Interruptions to maternal blood flow due to preexisting or chronic conditions can cause decreased cardiac output, which can lead to decreased oxygen in the maternal blood, which then causes decreased oxygenation of the fetus.

Nursing Interventions

- Assess patient via continuous EFM to observe and identify fetal response to any disruption of the maternal–fetal oxygen pathway.
- Implement nursing interventions to increase blood flow and promote fetal oxygenation: Reposition patient into a lateral position. Administer IV fluid bolus. Administer supplemental oxygen. Modify pushing efforts. Decrease oxytocin rate by decreasing oxytocin, removing prostaglandin E2 insert, and/or withholding next dose of misoprostol.

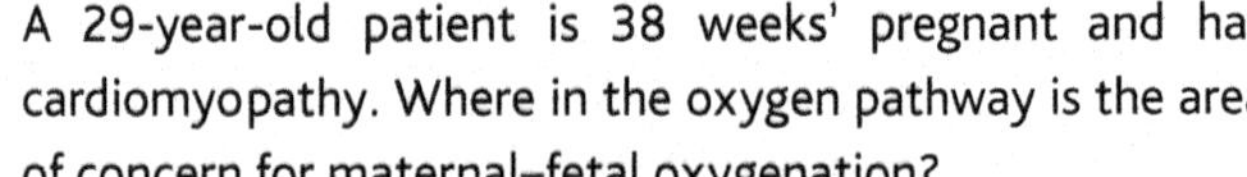

POP QUIZ 5.1

A 29-year-old patient is 38 weeks' pregnant and has cardiomyopathy. Where in the oxygen pathway is the area of concern for maternal–fetal oxygenation?

MATERNAL HYPOTENSION

- *Hypotension* is typically defined as maternal blood pressure (BP) of less than or equal to 90/60 mmHg.
- Causes of maternal hypotension include cardiac condition; dehydration; epidural or spinal anesthesia; excessive blood loss, hemorrhage, or hemorrhagic shock; supine position or inferior vena cava (IVC) syndrome.
- Hypotension interrupts the maternal–fetal oxygen pathway by reducing placental blood flow, perfusion, and exchange of gases.
- Anesthesia: Epidural or spinal anesthesia affects the nerve fibers that control muscle contractions inside the blood vessels, which causes the blood vessels to relax due to vasodilation, thereby lowering BP. The resulting hypotension can affect fetal oxygenation.

Nursing Interventions

- Call for additional assistance and notify provider.
- Maintain continuous monitoring of FHR tracing. The nurse may observe late decelerations; minimal or absent variability.
- Monitor maternal BP. ▶

Nursing Interventions (*continued*)

- Monitor patients with underlying heart conditions with continuous three-lead EKG.
- Reposition patient into left lateral position to increase blood flow back to uterus.
- Administer IV fluid bolus per order. May obtain additional IV access for blood administration if needed.
- Administer supplemental oxygen: Administer 10 L/min via nonrebreather face mask; discontinue as soon as possible based on fetal status.
- Anesthesia-specific nursing interventions: Epidural—notify provider and anesthesiologist of maternal hypotension and vital signs; anesthesiologist may administer ephedrine. Spinal—anesthesia team will manage hypotension in the operating room.

HYPERTENSIVE DISORDERS IN PREGNANCY

- Hypertensive disorders in pregnancy include disorders related to hypertension.
- Hypertensive disorders can be classified as chronic hypertension (not pregnancy related); eclampsia; gestational hypertension; HELLP syndrome (hemolysis, elevated liver enzymes, and low platelets); or preeclampsia, superimposed, with or without severe features.
- *Chronic hypertension* is defined as BP greater than or equal to 140 mmHg systolic and/or 90 mmHg diastolic before pregnancy or before 20 weeks of gestation.
- *Eclampsia* is defined by new-onset tonic-clonic, focal, or multifocal seizures in the absence of other causative conditions.
- *Gestational hypertension* is characterized by systolic BP of 140 mmHg or more or diastolic BP of 90 mmHg or more, or both, on two occasions at least 4 hours apart after 20 weeks of gestation.
- *HELLP syndrome* is diagnosed in patients with *h*emolysis, *e*levated *l*iver enzymes, and *l*ow *p*latelet count.
- *Preeclampsia* is associated with new-onset hypertension, which occurs most often after 20 weeks of gestation and often near term. Preeclampsia is often accompanied by new-onset proteinuria; it is often diagnosed with gestational hypertension and proteinuria (greater than or equal to 300 mg in 24-hour collection or a protein/creatinine ratio of greater than or equal to 0.3 mg/dL). Hypertension and other signs or symptoms of preeclampsia may present in some patients without proteinuria.
- *Gestational hypertension* in the absence of proteinuria is diagnosed with preeclampsia with severe features if any of the following are present: impaired liver function; new-onset headache; pulmonary edema; renal insufficiency; severe persistent right upper quadrant or epigastric pain; severe range BPs with systolic BP of 160 mmHg or higher or diastolic BP of 110 mmHg or higher; thrombocytopenia (platelet count less than 100,000); visual disturbances.
- Treatments include magnesium sulfate to prevent seizures; medications for severe range BPs (Table 5.1).

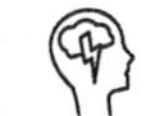

COMPLICATIONS

Complications for the fetus include fetal growth restriction and preterm birth. Complications to maternal body systems include cardiovascular effects, eclampsia, HELLP syndrome, liver damage, renal damage, retinal damage, placental abruption, pulmonary edema, and neurologic effects such as hypertensive encephalopathy. In addition, stroke is the leading cause of maternal morbidity from preeclampsia.

POP QUIZ 5.2

What is a possible diagnosis for a patient with new onset of seizures during pregnancy or the postpartum period without a preexisting neurologic disorder?

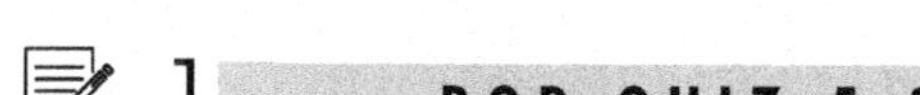

NURSING PEARL

Preeclampsia with severe features can cause pulmonary edema. Patients in labor sometimes receive large amounts of IV fluids. It is important to limit fluids for these patients to a total of 125 mL/hr (3,000 mL in 24 hours).

TABLE 5.1 Medications for Hypertension

INDICATIONS	MECHANISM OF ACTION	CONTRAINDICATIONS, PRECAUTIONS, AND ADVERSE EFFECTS
Anticonvulsant (magnesium sulfate)		
• Preeclampsia with severe features	• Relaxes smooth muscles to reduce chance of seizures	• Medication is contraindicated in patients with myasthenia gravis. • Side effects include flushing, nausea, diaphoresis, loss of deep tendon reflexes, respiratory depression, and cardiac arrest.
Antidotes (calcium gluconate)		
• Magnesium toxicity	• Direct antagonism of magnesium at the site of action	• There are no contraindications. • Administer slowly through IV push. • Side effects include syncope and bradycardia.
Beta-blockers (labetalol)		
• Hypertensive disorder	• Relax blood vessels and slow heart rate	• Medication is contraindicated in patients with asthma, atrioventricular heart block, and hypotension. • Side effects include lightheadedness, shortness of breath, low heart rate, and severe headache.
Calcium channel blockers (nifedipine)		
• Hypertensive disorder	• Relax muscles in heart	• Medication is contraindicated with hypotension and cardiac lesions. • Side effects include flushing, dizziness, hypotension, and slower heart rate.
Vasodilator (hydralazine)		
• Hypertensive disorder	• Relaxes muscles in blood vessels to help them dilate	• Medication is contraindicated in patients with coronary artery disease or rheumatic heart disease affecting the mitral valve. • Side effects include chest pain or pressure, light headed feeling, and numbness in hands and feet.

Causes

- May be indeterminate
- Possible risk factors: antiphospholipid antibody syndrome; assisted reproductive technology; chronic hypertension; gestational diabetes; maternal age 35 years or older; multifetal gestations; nulliparity; obstructive sleep apnea; preeclampsia in a previous pregnancy; pregestational diabetes; prepregnancy body mass index (BMI) greater than 30; renal disease; systemic lupus erythematosus; thrombophilia

Nursing Interventions

- Assess daily weight, input/output (I/O), and signs of edema.
- Monitor vital signs closely, specifically BP.
- Assess deep tendon reflexes.
- Assess lung sounds for signs of pulmonary edema.
- Assess for headache unrelieved by medication, level of consciousness, neurologic status for magnesium toxicity, and visual changes.
- Assess FHR.

MATERNAL HYPOVOLEMIA AND HEMORRHAGE

- *Maternal hypovolemia* is a decrease in the amount of circulating maternal blood volume.
- *Maternal hemorrhage* is the excessive loss of maternal blood.
- Causes of maternal hypovolemia include anemia and hemorrhage.
- Causes of maternal hemorrhage: placental abruption (see Placenta section); placenta previa; unrepaired laceration from delivery (postpartum hemorrhage [PPH] after delivery of fetus); uterine rupture (see Uterus section)
- Both hypovolemia and hemorrhage lead to reduced maternal cardiac output, affecting placental perfusion. This leads to decreased blood flow to the fetus and decreased fetal oxygenation.

Nursing Interventions

- If fetus is still in utero: Call for help. Monitor patient. Reposition patient into left lateral position. Administer IV fluid bolus. Administer supplemental oxygen. Measure blood loss; quantified blood loss (QBL) measurement is the preferred method. Notify provider and initiate OB rapid response team (if applicable or available). Prepare for administration of blood products. Prepare for emergent delivery. Call for help. Administer IV fluid bolus. Monitor maternal vital signs for tachycardia and hypotension. Initiate OB rapid response team (if available). Prepare for administration of blood products. Prepare to administer medications postpartum (Table 5.2). Weigh all pads and linens for accurate blood loss (1 mL = 1 g).

INFERIOR VENA CAVA COMPRESSION

- Compression of the maternal IVC, especially during active labor, contributes to decreased cardiac output and maternal hypotension due to decreased venous return and hypoperfusion.
- Compression of the IVC can be due to maternal supine positioning during late pregnancy. In supine position, the weight of the fetus and uterus can mechanically compress the IVC; this compression is referred to as *IVC syndrome*. ▶

[]   **ALERT!**

The antidote for magnesium sulfate is calcium gluconate administered via IV push over 5 to 10 minutes. This should always be available for any patient on magnesium sulfate. Toxicity symptoms include visual changes, flushing, muscle paralysis, and loss of deep tendon reflexes.

[ ] **POP QUIZ 5.3**

The nurse is strictly monitoring the patient's I/O and has advocated for the IV fluids not to be administered at a rate more than 125 mL/hr. What complication is the nurse trying to prevent?

[ ] **POP QUIZ 5.4**

A nurse is educating a pregnant patient on the risks of gestational hypertension. What symptoms could be mentioned?

[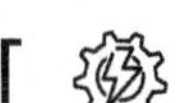]   **ALERT!**

A pregnant patient who is hemorrhaging needs immediate delivery and fluid volume replacement.

TABLE 5.2 Medications for Postpartum Hemorrhage

INDICATIONS	MECHANISM OF ACTION	CONTRAINDICATIONS, PRECAUTIONS, AND ADVERSE EFFECTS
Semisynthetic ergot alkaloid derivatives (methylergonovine maleate)		
• PPH	• Stimulate contraction of the uterus to prevent or stop hemorrhage	• Medication is contraindicated in patients with hypertension or in patients who are allergic. • Use caution in patients with sepsis. • Adverse effects include hypertension, headache, abdominal pain, nausea, and vomiting.
Prostaglandin F2-alpha analogue (carboprost tromethamine)		
• PPH	• Stimulates contraction of the uterus to prevent or stop hemorrhage	• Medication is contraindicated in patients with asthma; acute pelvic inflammatory disease; or active cardiac, pulmonary, renal, or hepatic disease, and in patients who are allergic. • Adverse effects include fever, vomiting, severe diarrhea, nausea, flushing, headaches, and cough.
Prostaglandin E1 analog (misoprostol)		
• PPH	• Stimulates contraction of the uterus to prevent or stop hemorrhage	• Medication is contraindicated in patients who are allergic. • Adverse effects include diarrhea, stomach pain, nausea, upset stomach, gas, and vaginal bleeding.
Cyclic nonapeptide hormone (oxytocin)		
• PPH	• Stimulates contraction of the uterus to prevent or stop hemorrhage	• Medication is contraindicated in patients who are allergic. • Adverse effects include nausea, vomiting, and more painful contractions.

PPH, postpartum hemorrhage.

INFERIOR VENA CAVA COMPRESSION (*continued*)

- A contributing factor of IVC syndrome is an enlarged uterus. Maternal symptoms include lightheadedness, nausea, dizziness, shortness of breath, hypotension, and tachycardia.
- EFM tracing may show late decelerations, variable decelerations, prolonged decelerations, minimal or absent variability, and fetal bradycardia.

Nursing Interventions

- Maintain continuous FHR tracing.
- Reposition patient to correct fetal decelerations. Left lateral position can relieve IVC compression, which will improve fetal oxygenation and FHR.
- Administer IV fluid bolus. ▶

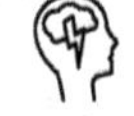

COMPLICATIONS

If not corrected, IVC compression can lead to decreased BP, thereby leading to late decelerations in the fetus and ultimately fetal death.

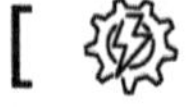

ALERT!

An FHR tracing that indicates inadequate fetal oxygenation is an urgent situation because it is unknown how long the fetus has not been receiving adequate oxygen. If FHR variability is absent, the patient must be evaluated by the provider urgently. Interventions to improve fetal oxygenation (IV fluid bolus, position change) should be implemented, and the fetus may need to be delivered by Cesarean section.

Nursing Interventions (*continued*)

- Administer supplemental oxygen: Administer 10 L/min via nonrebreather face mask; discontinue as soon as possible based on fetal status.
- Encourage modification of pushing efforts: Push with every second or every third contraction; push while lying on side; temporarily discontinue pushing (during second stage labor).
- Evaluate fetal response to interventions.

MATERNAL SEIZURE

- A *seizure* is a sudden, uncontrolled electrical disturbance in the brain.
- Seizures can cause changes in behavior, movements, feelings, and levels of consciousness.
- Two types of seizures are commonly seen during pregnancy: *focal*, which is abnormal activity in one area of brain; and *generalized*, which affects the entire brain.
- Maternal seizures can be harmful to the fetus due to the resulting increase in BP, decreased oxygenation, and electrolyte changes. The increase in intrauterine pressure during a seizure may also decrease uteroplacental blood flow.
- Causes: bleeding in the brain, brain tumor, eclampsia (seizure is possible when preeclampsia has progressed or is not controlled; preeclampsia can cause hypertension, proteinuria, hyperreflexia, headache, visual disturbances, and epigastric pain, and can progress to eclampsia), epilepsy, hypertension, stroke

Nursing Interventions

- Administer magnesium sulfate for eclamptic seizure (Table 5.3).
- Administer medication to treat severe hypertension in patients with preeclampsia (see Table 5.1): hydralazine, nifedipine
- Maintain continuous monitoring of FHR; may observe late decelerations, minimal or absent variability
- Keep patient safe: Monitor vital signs for return to baseline. Monitor neurologic status until returned to baseline. Use padded side rails. Remain with patient.

UTERUS

UTERINE RUPTURE

- *Uterine rupture* is a spontaneous tear in the uterus.
- Uterine rupture can cause massive maternal hemorrhage and severe fetal distress. Uterine arteries may bleed out of uterus into abdomen. Fetus can move out of uterus into abdomen.
- Causes of uterine rupture: excessive use of uterotonics; overdistention of uterus; multifetal pregnancy; polyhydramnios; external cephalic version; trial of labor after Cesarean section.

Nursing Interventions

- Maintain continuous FHR tracing. May observe bradycardia; prolonged deceleration, late decelerations, or sinusoidal pattern; minimal variability or absent variability. ▶

[📝] POP QUIZ 5.5

What are the risks associated with a pregnant patient lying in the supine position during the later weeks of the third trimester of pregnancy?

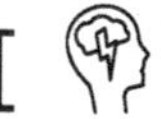

COMPLICATIONS

If not corrected, IVC compression can lead to decreased BP, thereby leading to late decelerations in the fetus and ultimately fetal death.

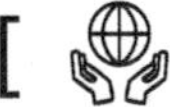

NURSING PEARL

Uteroplacental issues cause late decelerations.

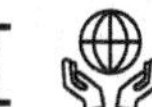

NURSING PEARL

Always maintain clear, closed-loop communication with the OB team and providers when providing maternal stabilization.

TABLE 5.3 Medications for Preterm Labor

INDICATIONS	MECHANISM OF ACTION	CONTRAINDICATIONS, PRECAUTIONS, AND ADVERSE EFFECTS
Anticonvulsant (magnesium sulfate)		
• Neuroprotection in preterm neonate	Exact mechanism unknown, but thought to: • Protect against inflammatory and oxidative injury • Stabilize BP and normalize cerebral blood flow • Stabilize neuronal membranes and block excitatory neurotransmitters	• Medication is contraindicated in patients with myasthenia gravis. • Adverse effects include flushing, nausea, diaphoresis, loss of deep tendon reflexes, respiratory depression, and cardiac arrest.
Beta-adrenergic receptor agonists (isoproterenol, ritodrine)		
• Preterm labor	• Inhibit uterine contractions	• Medication is contraindicated in patients with tachycardia-sensitive cardiac disease and poorly controlled diabetes mellitus. • Adverse effects include tachycardia, hypotension, tremors, palpitations, shortness of breath, and chest pain.
Calcium channel blockers (nifedipine)		
• Preterm labor	• Relax the muscles in the uterus	• Medication is contraindicated in patients with hypotension and cardiac lesions. • Adverse effects include flushing, dizziness, hypotension, and slower heart rate.
Corticosteroid (betamethasone)		
• Lung maturity	• Causes release of surfactant	• Medication can increase blood sugar.
NSAID (indomethacin)		
• Preterm labor	• Blocks the production of prostaglandin, which causes contractions	• Medication is contraindicated in patients with platelet or bleeding disorders. • Adverse effects include nausea, vomiting, and reflux.

BP, blood pressure; NSAID, nonsteroidal anti-inflammatory drug.

Nursing Interventions (*continued*)

- Discontinue oxytocin, if applicable.
- Notify provider.
- Prepare for emergent Cesarean section.
- Prepare for PPH after delivery.
- Prepare to administer postpartum medications (see Table 5.2): methylergonovine maleate, carboprost tromethamine, misoprostol, oxytocin, tranexamic acid

[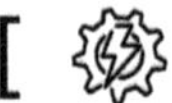]   **ALERT!**

If a patient is pushing and the head is at +3 station and then suddenly goes back to −1 station, call provider immediately due to symptoms of uterine rupture.

EXCESSIVE UTERINE ACTIVITY (TACHYSYSTOLE)

- *Excessive uterine activity*, also known as *tachysystole*, is defined as more than five contractions in 10 minutes.
- Excessive uterine activity causes *increased uterine resting tone*, which is pressure within the uterus when it is not contracting. This can impair placental circulation and lead to decreased FHR variability.
- When excessive uterine activity occurs, the FHR may show minimal, late, variable, or prolonged decelerations. Figure 5.1 shows an FHR tracing demonstrating variable decelerations with absent to minimal variability; note the frequency of the uterine contractions.
- Causes of excessive uterine activity are unknown, but may include cervical ripening agents, chorioamnionitis, maternal dehydration, oxytocin, placental abruption, or uterine rupture.

Nursing Interventions

- Maintain continuous monitoring of FHR tracing; may observe late, variable, or prolonged decelerations.
- Decrease or discontinue oxytocin if it is being administered.
- Administer supplemental oxygen: Administer 10 L/min via nonrebreather face mask; discontinue as soon as possible based on fetal status.
- Administer tocolytics per order, with the objectives of returning uterine activity to normal spacing of contractions and decreasing the uterine resting tone to the normal range.
- Administer IV fluid bolus or increase IV fluid rate per order.

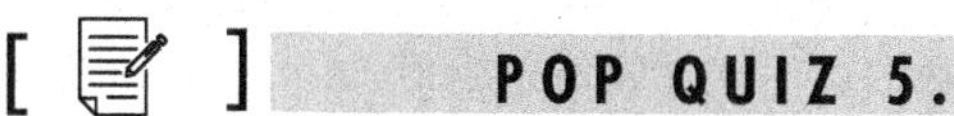

POP QUIZ 5.6

A 34-year-old patient gave birth to her fifth baby 2 hours ago and has not been able to void since delivery. The patient calls for help because she passed a large egg-sized clot and is still leaking blood. An assessment finds a boggy fundus, but it is located +2 and to the right. What is the likely cause and the appropriate intervention?

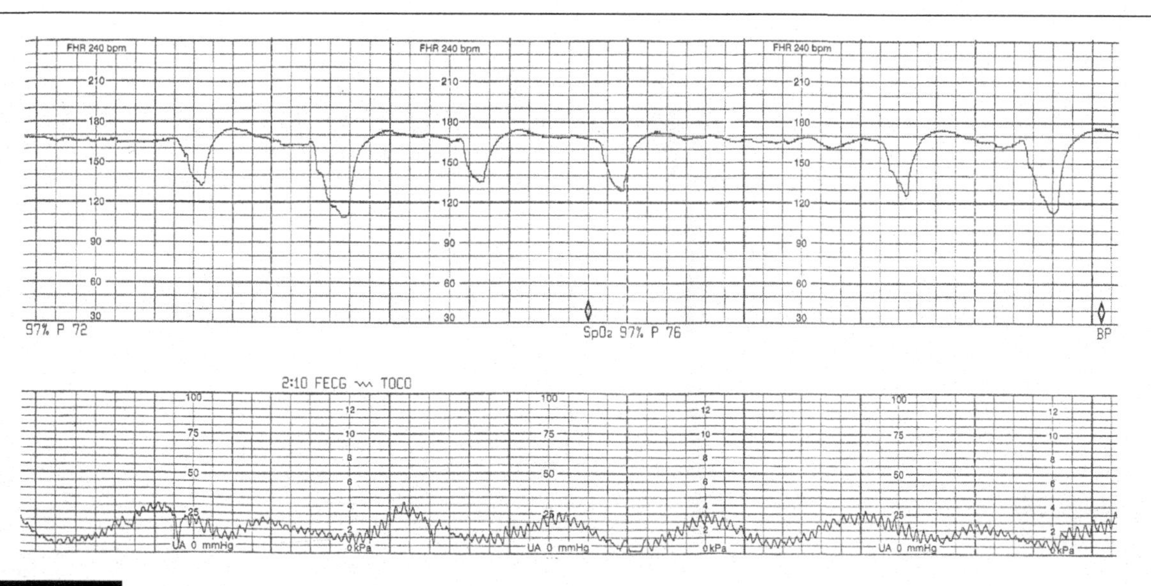

FIGURE 5.1 Excessive uterine activity with variable decelerations.

Source: Murray, M., Huelsmann, G., & Koperski, N. (2019). *Essentials of fetal and uterine monitoring* (5th ed.). Springer Publishing Company.

PLACENTA

ABRUPTIO PLACENTAE

- *Abruptio placentae* is the complete or partial separation of the placenta from the uterine wall. Partial (chronic) separation may be able to stabilize without complications. Complete separation requires emergent delivery.
- Abruptio placentae compromises fetal oxygenation due to collapse or destruction of the intervillous space and interference with the fetal supply of oxygen and nutrients.
- Abruptio placentae can be reflected on FHR tracing by a sinusoidal FHR pattern, which reflects fetal compromise from decreased oxygenation (Figure 5.2).
- Causes of abruption include abdominal trauma, cocaine use, high BP, and preeclampsia and eclampsia.
- Symptoms include heavy vaginal bleeding, hypotension, maternal tachycardia, severe abdominal pain, and rigid abdomen.

[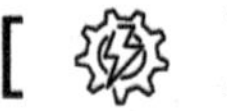]   **ALERT!**

Diabetes affects the development of and the function of the placenta. Nurses should be aware that maternal blood sugar may need to be assessed.

Nursing Interventions

- Call for help.
- Monitor blood loss. If patient is visibly bleeding, measure pads and linens for accurate blood loss (1 mL = 1 g).
- Monitor vital signs for signs of shock, including tachycardia and hypotension.
- Maintain continuous FHR tracing; may observe late or prolonged decelerations or sinusoidal pattern, bradycardia, or minimal or absent FHR variability. ▶

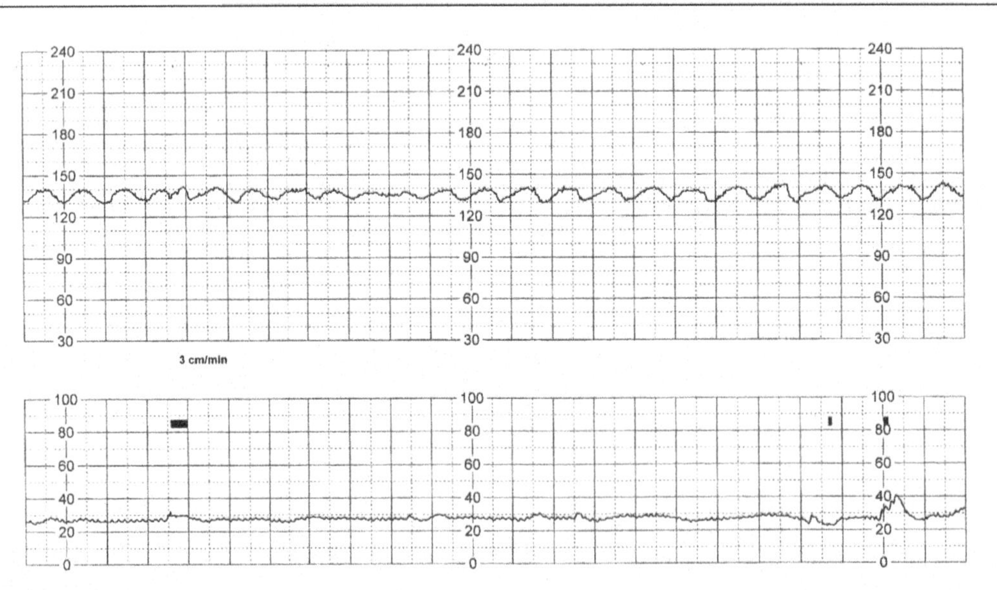

FIGURE 5.2   This FHR tracing is from a 29-year-old patient being evaluated after a motor vehicle crash. The patient's abdomen is hard and painful, and the patient is experiencing vaginal bleeding. This tracing is a sinusoidal pattern, likely due to a placental abruption caused by the motor vehicle crash.

FHR, fetal heart rate.

Source: Murray, M., Huelsmann, G., & Koperski, N. (2019). *Essentials of fetal and uterine monitoring* (5th ed.). Springer Publishing Company.

Nursing Interventions (*continued*)

- Reposition patient to left lateral position.
- Obtain IV access and administer IV fluid bolus.
- Administer supplemental oxygen: Administer 10 L/min via nonrebreather face mask; discontinue as soon as possible based on fetal status.
- Collect blood for complete blood count (CBC) and type and screen lab tests.
- Prepare for possible emergent delivery.

PLACENTAL IMPLANTATION COMPLICATIONS

- Placenta accreta is a serious complication and occurs when the placenta implants too deeply into the uterus.
- Placenta increta invades the muscles of the uterus, and placenta percreta grows through the uterine wall. These complications will require Cesarean section to deliver fetus and possible hysterectomy.

Causes and Risk Factors

- Advanced maternal age
- Previous childbirth (increased risk with each delivery)
- Previous uterine surgery

Nursing Interventions

- Prepare for blood transfusion.
- Prepare for Cesarean section and possible hysterectomy.
- Provide emotional support.

UMBILICAL CORD

NUCHAL CORD

- Nuchal cord occurs when the umbilical cord wraps around the fetus's neck while in utero.
- The umbilical cord may be loosely or tightly wrapped around the fetus's neck one or more times.
- Complications are more likely to occur if the nuchal cord is tight.
- Nuchal cord can be an incidental finding at birth.
- Nuchal cord can cause recurrent variable decelerations.

Causes

- Fetal size or movements: small preterm fetus; fetus that flipped from breech to vertex
- Possible differential flow patterns in umbilical cord

Nursing Interventions

- Monitor fetus using continuous EFM.
- Perform interventions related to FHR tracing, if indicated (Figure 5.3): Change patient position. Administer IV fluid bolus. Administer oxygen. Notify provider. Prepare for Cesarean section delivery, if required.

POP QUIZ 5.7

A 19-year-old patient presents to labor and delivery (L&D) in excruciating abdominal pain with a large amount of bright-red vaginal bleeding and appears to be pregnant and close to full term. The patient has not had prenatal care. What is an appropriate assessment, and what nursing interventions are needed?

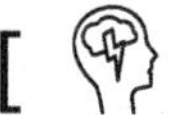

COMPLICATIONS

Up to 20% of fetal demise autopsies demonstrate fatal compromise of umbilical cord circulation.

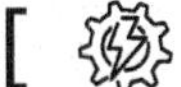

ALERT!

Cord compression and umbilical cord prolapse can also cause variable decelerations.

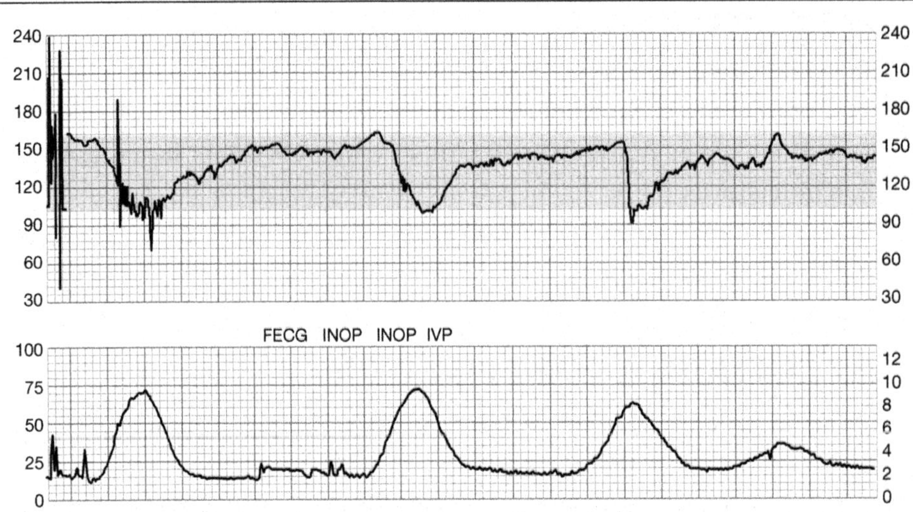

FIGURE 5.3   FHR showing a possible nuchal cord. This is a category II FHR with a baseline of 150 bpm, moderate variability, no accelerations, and variable decelerations.

bpm, beats per minute; FHR, fetal heart rate.

Source: Nye, R. (2019). *Essentials of fetal heart rate monitoring.* Springer Publishing Company.

UMBILICAL CORD COMPRESSION

- *Umbilical cord compression* is mechanical pressure on the umbilical cord from the fetus.
- Umbilical cord compression induces fetal baroceptor stimulation and parasympathetic response, causing variable decelerations in the FHR, as well as minimal or absent variability.
- Umbilical cord compression can be caused by the cord wrapped around fetal body; cord wrapped around fetal neck; fetus holding onto the cord; oligohydramnios; position of fetus.
- Umbilical cord compression causes a transient disruption of the maternal–fetal oxygen pathway and can block blood flow.

[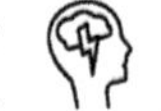]   **COMPLICATIONS**

If compression or a blood clot blocks the umbilical vein, the fetus could suffer permanent injury or even death.

Nursing Interventions

- Maintain continuous FHR tracing; may observe variable decelerations (Figure 5.4).
- Reposition patient to correct variable decelerations and relieve cord compression: hands and knees position; left or right lateral position
- Administer IV fluid bolus.
- Administer supplemental oxygen: Administer 10 L/min via nonrebreather face mask; discontinue as soon as possible based on fetal status.
- Encourage modification of pushing efforts during labor: pushing with every other or every third contraction; pushing on side; temporary discontinuation of pushing.
- Evaluate fetal response to interventions.
- Prepare for amnioinfusion: *Amnioinfusion* is a treatment for persistent variable decelerations in the presence of ruptured membranes. Amnioinfusion is used to increase fluid volume via the infusion of normal sterile saline through the cervix. Observe for fluid return from the vagina on the underpad. Fluid that is administered must be discharged from the vagina. If there is no fluid return, turn off amnioinfusion to prevent uterine rupture.

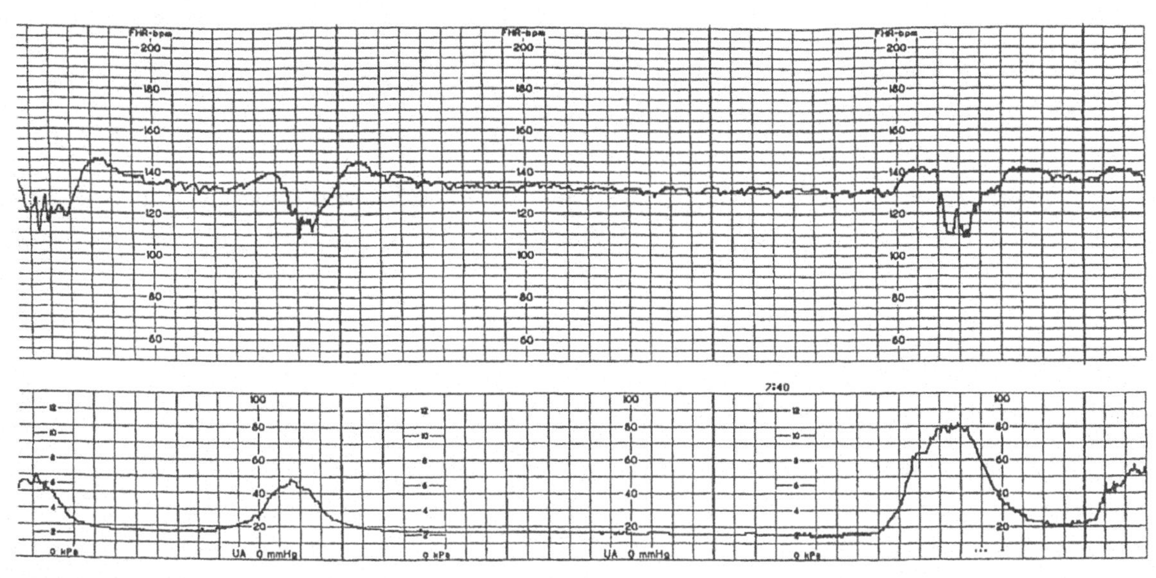

FIGURE 5.4   Variable decelerations.

Source: Murray, M., Huelsmann, G., & Koperski, N. (2019). *Essentials of fetal and uterine monitoring* (5th ed.). Springer Publishing Company.

UMBILICAL CORD PROLAPSE

- *Umbilical cord prolapse* occurs when the umbilical cord enters the birth canal through the cervix ahead of the fetus.
- A prolapsed cord can cause obstruction of blood flow through the umbilical cord, which can affect fetal oxygenation and fetal blood flow.
- Umbilical cord prolapse is indicated when the cord can be seen or palpated on examination.
- FHR tracing may show fetal bradycardia or variable or prolonged decelerations.
- Causes of umbilical cord prolapse: rupture of membranes before 32 weeks' gestation; premature, artificial, or spontaneous rupture of membranes; greater or equal to 4 cm cervical dilation; higher fetal station in which the fetal head is not well engaged in the pelvic inlet; malpresentation of fetus (e.g., breech or transverse position).

[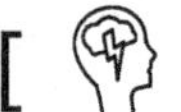]   **COMPLICATIONS**

Umbilical cord prolapse causes mechanical cord compression due to pressure from the fetus and stretching of the cord, leading to compromised fetal oxygen supply.

Nursing Interventions

- Maintain continuous monitoring of FHR tracing.
- Assess for pulsating umbilical cord presence in vagina.
- Reposition and elevate fetus off the cord manually.
- Reposition patient in Trendelenburg position.
- Notify provider and prepare for emergent operative delivery (Cesarean section).

FETUS

HYPOXIA/ACIDOSIS

- Hypoxia occurs prior to labor or during L&D when the following occurs: Fetal oxygen is impaired. A persistent category II FHR tracing, lasting longer than 60 minutes with minimal or absent variability, indicates possible hypoxia. A category I tracing changes to category III, which is indicative of an acute hypoxic event (Figure 5.5).
- Acidosis occurs with excessive buildup of hydrogen in tissues. Acidosis is caused by fetal hypoxia and can cause long-term morbidity.

Causes and Risk Factors

- Maternal cigarette smoking
- Fetal anemia
- Maternal cardiovascular disease
- Maternal respiratory condition
- Placental abruption
- Placental infarction
- Preeclampsia
- Prolapsed or occluded umbilical cord

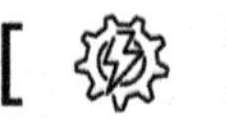

[⚡]   ALERT!

During an umbilical cord prolapse, the nurse may observe variable or prolonged decelerations or fetal bradycardia.

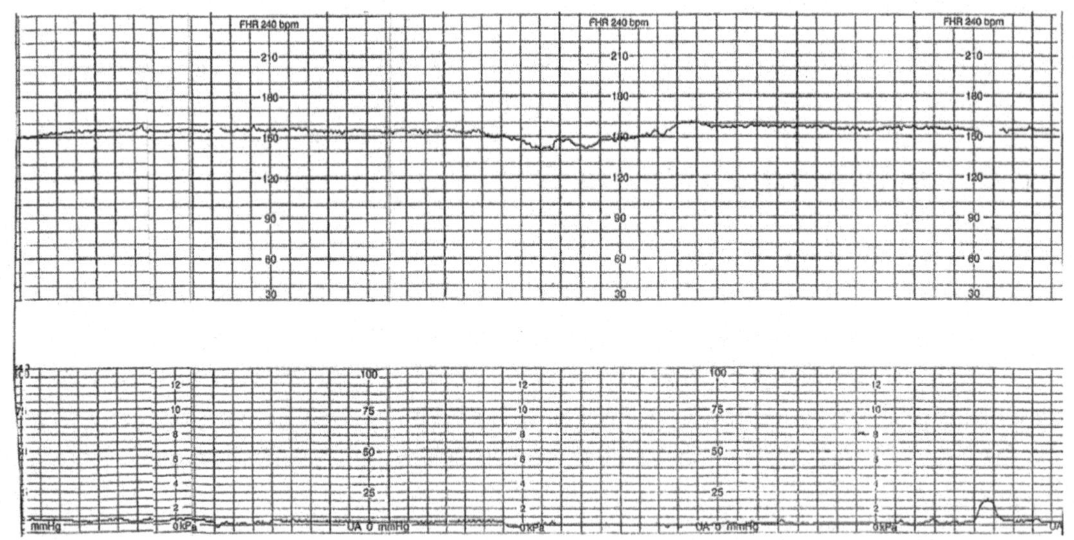

FIGURE 5.5   FHR with absent variability, a spontaneous deceleration, and no accelerations demonstrates fetal hypoxia. This is a category III FHR that needs immediate interventions. The nurse should call the provider, get help to start an IV and give IV fluid bolus, reposition the patient, and administer oxygen.

bpm, beats per minute; FHR, fetal heart rate.

Source: Murray, M., Huelsmann, G., & Koperski, N. (2019). *Essentials of fetal and uterine monitoring* (5th ed.). Springer Publishing Company.

Nursing Interventions

- Monitor fetus using continuous EFM.
- Perform interventions if category II or III FHR tracing: Change patient position; administer IV fluid bolus; administer oxygen 8 to 10 L per mask; notify provider; prepare for Cesarean section delivery, if required.
- Obtain a cord blood gas sample from the umbilical cord: Collect from umbilical artery (UA) first, then umbilical vein (UV). Difference in artery and vein gases may give further information on duration. Results show fetal oxygenation status at time of delivery. Results can help the neonatal care team to understand the effectiveness of organ function and the ability of the baby to compensate for acute or chronic changes at the moment of birth.

SHOULDER DYSTOCIA

- *Shoulder dystocia* occurs when one or both fetal shoulders are impacted behind the symphysis pubis, or when descent of the fetal shoulder is obstructed by the sacral promontory after delivery of head.
- Shoulder dystocia results in prolonged delivery; the time from delivery of head to delivery of body is more than 60 seconds.

Causes and Risk Factors

- May be indeterminate
- Larger than average fetus (greater than 4,000 g)
- Maternal risk factors: abnormal pelvic anatomy; advanced age; diabetes; macrosomic fetus; multiparity; obesity and excessive gestational weight gain; postterm pregnancy; previous shoulder dystocia; short stature

Nursing Interventions

- Prepare to have extra nurses present at delivery if a large fetus (greater than 4,000 g) is expected based on ultrasound or Leopold's maneuver.
- Prepare for delivery with resuscitation equipment and appropriate personnel for neonate.
- Stay calm.
- Assist provider with maneuvers. Primary maneuvers: McRoberts maneuver and suprapubic pressure. Secondary maneuvers: Gaskin maneuver, posterior axilla sling traction, Rubin maneuver, Woods screw maneuver (all except Gaskin maneuver are performed by provider). Desperation maneuvers: intentional breaking of fetal clavicle, Zavanelli maneuver (these are performed by provider as last attempt, due to increased risk of maternal and fetal morbidity and mortality).
- Ensure that all maneuvers performed are included in delivery documentation.

[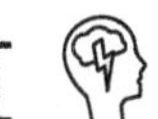]　**ALERT!**

Cord blood gases (UA and UV) can help to determine whether the hypoxia is occurring before or during labor.

[]　**COMPLICATIONS**

In the neonate, brachial plexus injury and clavicle and humerus fractures are possible. Hypoxic ischemic brain injury or death can occur. In the patient, vaginal lacerations, uterine rupture, or PPH can occur.

[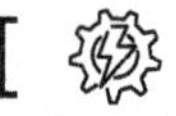]　**ALERT!**

A prolonged second stage of labor may be predictive of a shoulder dystocia and should alert the nurse to have extra help available.

[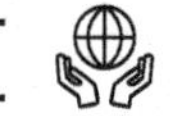]　**ALERT!**

The turtle sign (fetal head, usually dark red or purple, appearing and retracting during pushing) suggests a possible shoulder dystocia.

[   ]　**NURSING PEARL**

The key to managing complications is to be prepared. Practice for emergencies by performing simulation drills. When complications occur, remain calm and get help.

OTHER MATERNAL COMPLICATIONS

CHORIOAMNIONITIS

- *Chorioamnionitis* is an infection of the amniotic sac, most often bacterial in origin.
- Chorioamnionitis occurs in about 4% of deliveries at term but occurs more frequently in preterm deliveries and with premature rupture of membranes.
- A major risk factor for chorioamnionitis is prolonged rupture of membranes.
- Signs and symptoms: fetal tachycardia, foul-smelling amniotic fluid, maternal fever, uterine tenderness
- Chorioamnionitis is a risk factor for both maternal and neonatal sequelae.
- Neonatal complications: bronchopulmonary dysplasia in premature infants, cerebral palsy, neonatal death, neonatal sepsis, neurologic abnormalities, premature birth, respiratory distress syndrome, retinopathy of prematurity
- Maternal complications: maternal sepsis, operative delivery, PPH, preterm delivery, severe pelvic infections, subcutaneous wound infections

Causes

- Existing infection such as *Candida*, *Escherichia coli*, group B *Streptococcus*, trichomoniasis
- Multiple vaginal examinations after rupture of membranes
- Prolonged rupture of membranes

Nursing Interventions

- Administer antibiotics and antipyretics as ordered.
- Monitor maternal temperature frequently, per institutional policy.
- Use continuous fetal monitoring to assess for FHR complications.
- Send placenta cultures to lab after delivery, as ordered by provider.

POSTPARTUM HEMORRHAGE

- PPH is characterized as a cumulative blood loss of 1,000 mL or more after delivery.
- Measuring blood loss is a key component of recognizing PPH; estimation is inaccurate.
- PPH may occur immediately after birth or up to 12 weeks after delivery.
- PPH needs immediate intervention and treatment.
- Medications used for PPH (see Table 5.2): carboprost tromethamine, methylergonovine maleate, misoprostol, oxytocin, tranexamic acid
- Other treatments include blood replacement; emptying of bladder; fundal massage; IV fluid replacement; removal of retained placenta; repair of lacerations; surgical interventions (hysterectomy, uterine artery embolization, uterine compression sutures).

[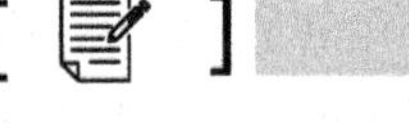]   **POP QUIZ 5.8**

A 37-year-old patient with gestational diabetes is in L&D for induction of labor due to uncontrolled blood sugars. Height is 4'10, and weight is 220 lb. The abdomen appears large. The patient is 10 cm dilated and starts pushing. What should the nurse caring for this patient do?

[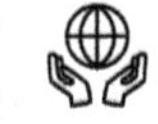]   **NURSING PEARL**

Use a "bundle" that helps to recognize and treat PPH. Evidence-based patient safety bundles provide algorithms and instructions for caring for a patient who is hemorrhaging.

[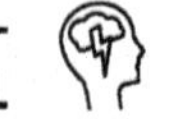]   **COMPLICATIONS**

PPH can be life threatening and needs immediate attention.

Causes and Risk Factors

- Atony of the uterus, which may be due to numerous risk factors: distended (full) bladder, infection, large fetus, medication (use of magnesium sulfate or prolonged use of oxytocin), multiparous patient, multiple gestation
- Bleeding or clotting disorder; may not be diagnosed prior to giving birth
- Retained tissue: Placental fragments or amniotic membrane remain in uterus; small placental fragments can lead to delayed PPH.
- Trauma: hematoma (collection of blood can occur from forceps or vacuum use); lacerations of the vagina or cervix that are not completely repaired can continue to bleed, leading to hemorrhage.

Nursing Interventions

- Administer medications as ordered.
- Administer oxygen if needed.
- Apply Foley or straight catheter if needed.
- Assist with tamponade insertion if used.
- Request assistance from additional nurses and provider and assign roles.
- Measure QBL: Weigh pads and linens. Subtract dry weight from blood-soaked weight to calculate QBL; 1g = 1 mL blood.
- Perform fundal checks for uterine tone after delivery per protocol.
- When observing blood loss, always roll the patient and check for pooled blood under the buttocks.
- Perform fundal massage.
- Prepare patient for operating room as necessary.
- Provide an IV fluid bolus.
- Remain with the patient.

[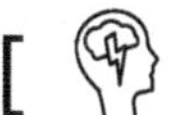]   **COMPLICATIONS**

PPH is the leading cause of maternal mortality in the world. Early recognition is imperative.

[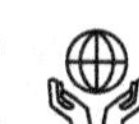]   **NURSING PEARL**

During fundal checks, the fundus should continue to contract and be felt at the same location or lower. If the fundal height increases or is palpated to the left or right (instead of midline), a full bladder should be suspected. The patient should void or may require catheterization.

DIABETES MELLITUS

- Two types of diabetes mellitus can be seen during pregnancy: gestational diabetes mellitus (GDM), which develops during pregnancy; pregestational diabetes mellitus, type 1 or type 2.
- Diabetes can cause increased risk of spontaneous abortion, congenital defects, and stillbirth. Increased fetal surveillance is necessary.

Causes and Risk Factors

- Pregestational: Type 1—family history. Type 2—age older than 45 years; family history; GDM during previous pregnancy; African American, Hispanic/Latinx, American Indian, or Alaska Native descent; obesity; physically active less than three times per week.
- GDM: age older than 25 years; family history of type 2 diabetes mellitus; African American, Hispanic/Latinx, American Indian, Alaska Native, Native Hawaiian, or Pacific Islander descent; GDM during previous pregnancy; has given birth to baby over 9 lb; history of polycystic ovary syndrome; obesity.

Nursing Interventions

- Monitor maternal blood sugars per hospital policy.
- Monitor fetal status per hospital policy.

OBESITY

- Obesity is characterized by a BMI that is 30 or higher.
- Maternal obesity may be associated with certain conditions in the fetus: birth defects, childhood asthma, childhood obesity, or macrosomia.
- Maternal complications of obesity may include GDM, hypertension (and preeclampsia), miscarriage, sleep apnea, and Cesarean section with risk of Cesarean section complications, such as wound infections.

Causes

- Genetics
- Thyroid disease
- Dietary habits

Nursing Interventions

- Educate patient about weight gain early in pregnancy.
- No interventions are provided in L&D.

COMPLICATIONS OF LABOR

For normal uterine activity, see the end of Chapter 4.

FAILURE TO PROGRESS

- *Failure to progress* is defined as: active labor (greater than or equal to 6 cm dilated) after rupture of membranes, but with no cervical change after 4 hours of adequate uterine contractions; rupture of membranes but no cervical change after 6 hours of inadequate contractions with use of oxytocin.
- *Prolonged latent phase of labor* (less than 6 cm dilated) is defined as more than 20 hours for a primiparous patient or more than 14 hours for a multiparous patient.
- *Arrest of labor in second stage* is defined as multiparous patient pushing for at least 2 hours or primiparous patient pushing for at least 3 hours.

Causes

- Excessive maternal weight gain
- Induction of labor
- Macrosomic fetus
- Malpresentation of fetus
- Psychological issues (stress, anxiety, fear)
- Small maternal pelvis

Nursing Interventions

- Assist provider with manual fetal rotation.
- Assist provider with operative vaginal delivery.
- Provide continuous labor support.

OPERATIVE DELIVERY

- *Cesarean section* is operative delivery through surgical incision in the patient's abdomen. There is an increased risk of maternal morbidity due to possible hemorrhage; infection; placental complications with future pregnancies.
- *Operative vaginal delivery* is delivery with use of forceps or vacuum. There is a lower risk of maternal complications than with Cesarean section. Complications for neonate are not greater than those with Cesarean section.

Causes

- Failure to progress
- Macrosomic infant
- Malpresentation of fetus
- Maternal infection
- Multiple gestation
- Nonreassuring FHR

Nursing Interventions

- Assist provider as needed.
- Prepare patient for operative vaginal delivery. Instruct patient to listen to provider and push when directed.
- Prepare patient for Cesarean section: For abdominal prep remove hair with hair clippers. Clean skin according to institutional protocol. Provide emotional support. Obtain IV access. Move patient to operating room when ready.

PRETERM LABOR

- *Preterm labor* is defined as birth between 20 0/7 weeks of gestation and 36 6/7 weeks of gestation.
- It is the leading cause of neonatal mortality and the most common reason for antenatal hospitalization.

Causes and Risk Factors

- Age younger than 17 or older than 35 years
- Alcohol use
- Cigarette smoking
- Diabetes
- Drug use
- History of preterm birth
- Hypertensive disorders
- Infection: amniotic fluid, lower genital tract
- Interval of less than 6 months between pregnancies
- In vitro fertilization
- Multiple gestation
- Stressful events
- Trauma
- Uterus, cervix, or placenta problems

Nursing Interventions

- Administer medication as ordered.
- Treatment: A single course of corticosteroids is recommended for pregnant patients between 24 and 34 weeks of gestation who are at risk of delivery within 7 days. First-line tocolytic treatment with beta-adrenergic receptor agonists, calcium channel blockers, or nonsteroidal anti-inflammatory drugs (NSAIDs) for short-term prolongation of pregnancy (see Table 5.3). Tocolytic therapy to possibly prolong pregnancy long enough to administer antenatal corticosteroids and magnesium sulfate for neuroprotection.
- Educate patient on recognizing signs of preterm labor.
- Monitor FHR and contractions.

RESOURCES

American College of Obstetricians and Gynecologists. (2014a). Executive summary: Neonatal encephalopathy and neurologic outcome, second edition. *Obstetrics & Gynecology, 123*(4), 896–901. https://doi.org/10.1097/01.aog.0000445580.65983.d2

American College of Obstetricians and Gynecologists. (2014b). Obstetric Care Consensus No. 1: Safe prevention of the primary cesarean delivery. *Obstetrics & Gynecology, 123*(3), 693–711. https://doi.org/10.1097/01.aog.0000444441.04111.1d

American College of Obstetricians and Gynecologists. (2016). Practice Bulletin No. 171: Management of preterm labor. *Obstetrics & Gynecology, 128*(4), e155–e164. https://doi.org/10.1097/aog.0000000000001711

American College of Obstetricians and Gynecologists. (2017). Practice Bulletin No. 183: Postpartum hemorrhage. *Obstetrics & Gynecology, 130*(4), e168–e186. https://doi.org/10.1097/aog.0000000000002351

American College of Obstetricians and Gynecologists. (2018a). ACOG Practice Bulletin No. 190: Gestational diabetes mellitus. *Obstetrics & Gynecology, 131*(2), e49–e64. https://doi.org/10.1097/aog.0000000000002501

American College of Obstetricians and Gynecologists. (2018b). ACOG Practice Bulletin No. 201 summary: Pregestational diabetes mellitus. *Obstetrics & Gynecology, 132*(6), 1514–1516. https://doi.org/10.1097/aog.0000000000002961

American College of Obstetricians and Gynecologists. (2020). Gestational hypertension and preeclampsia. *Obstetrics & Gynecology, 135*(6), e237–e260. https://doi.org/10.1097/aog.0000000000003891

Conde-Agudelo, A., Romero, R., Jung, E. J., & Garcia Sánchez, Á. J. (2020). Management of clinical chorioamnionitis: An evidence-based approach. *American Journal of Obstetrics & Gynecology, 223*(6), 848–869. https://doi.org/10.1016/j.ajog.2020.09.044

Holland, T. (2020). Shoulder dystocia. *Nursing Made Incredibly Easy! 18*(6), 9–14. https://doi.org/10.1097/01.nme.0000717680.73079.f8

Mayo Foundation for Medical Education and Research. (2020a). *Placenta accreta.* https://www.mayoclinic.org/diseases-conditions/placenta-accreta/symptoms-causes/syc-20376431

Mayo Foundation for Medical Education and Research. (2020b). *Placental abruption.* https://www.mayoclinic.org/diseases-conditions/placental-abruption/symptoms-causes/syc-20376458

Moldenhauer, J. S. (2020). *Uterine rupture.* Merck Manuals Professional Version. https://www.merckmanuals.com/professional/gynecology-and-obstetrics/abnormalities-and-complications-of-labor-and-delivery/uterine-rupture

Murray, M., Huelsmann, G., & Koperski, N. (2019). *Essentials of fetal and uterine monitoring* (5th ed.). Springer Publishing Company.

National Institute for Health and Care Excellence. (2019). *Hypertension in pregnancy: Diagnosis and management.* https://www.nice.org.uk/guidance/ng133

Nye, R. (2019). *Essentials of fetal heart rate monitoring.* Springer Publishing Company.

Peesay, M. (2017). Nuchal cord and its implications. *Maternal Health, Neonatology and Perinatology, 3*(1), Article 28. https://doi.org/10.1186/s40748-017-0068-7

Prescribers' Digital Reference. (n.d.). *Invanz [Drug information].* https://www.pdr.net/drug-information/invanz?druglabelid=359

Sayed Ahmed, W. A., & Hamdy, M. A. (2018). Optimal management of umbilical cord prolapse. *International Journal of Women's Health, 10,* 459–465. https://doi.org/10.2147/IJWH.S130879

OVERVIEW

Ethical and legal issues, along with patient safety and quality improvement (QI), have important implications in obstetric nursing. This chapter covers these key points:

- Ethical decision-making plays a role in the care of the pregnant patient and fetus.
- Legal implications affect the care of the patient and fetus. Obstetrics is a high-risk, high-liability area of nursing and medicine.
- The safety of the patient and fetus must always be considered a priority.
- QI is an ongoing process to improve care for the patient.

ETHICS

Overview

- Four principles are used to address ethical issues, problems, and dilemmas: beneficence, justice, nonmaleficence, and respect for patient autonomy.
- *Beneficence* is doing good and providing care that benefits the patient. *Example:* The nurse who is caring for a patient in labor provides a massage to help with pain management.
- *Justice* is the principle of rendering to others what is due to them. *Example:* The medical staff uses a triage system to determine which patient receives care first.
- *Nonmaleficence* is an obligation to not cause harm or injury. *Example:* If a nurse is working while impaired, it is the responsibility of any nurse working with the impaired nurse to report them.
- *Respect for patient autonomy* acknowledges an individual's right to hold views, to make choices, and to act based on their own personal values and beliefs. Respect for autonomy provides a foundation for informed consent. Informed consent requires that staff adequately inform patients about their medical condition and the available therapies. Informed consent must be obtained by the provider with a witness present during the time of the consent and the patient signature. Respect for patient autonomy must consider the pregnant patient and the fetus (or fetuses), which may present conflicts between or among ethical principles.

Nursing Interventions

- Advocate for the patient.
- Contact hospital chaplain/clergy for spiritual care, as appropriate.
- Escalate to the ethics committee as needed.
- Follow the institution's policies and procedures.
- Provide emotional support to the patient and family members.
- Recognize signs and symptoms of moral distress. ▶

Nursing Interventions (*continued*)

- Report unethical and unsafe situations.
- Use the chain of command in situations when caring for a patient causes an ethical issue.
- Participate in code/event debrief to share experiences and identify opportunities for improvement.
- Review organizational guidelines for situations involving the nurse's personal or professional values (conscientious objection) in the care of maternal and neonatal complications.

POP QUIZ 6.1

A nurse is caring for a patient who has developed a birth plan that includes delayed bathing of the neonate. The nurse tells the patient that they cannot follow the birth plan because they need to bathe the newborn right away. What ethical principle applies to this situation?

POP QUIZ 6.2

An nurse volunteers at a clinic for underserved patients. What ethical principle is the nurse following?

LEGALITY

Overview

- Obstetrics is a high-litigation specialty.
- Complications leading to injury or death of a pregnant patient and/or a fetus may lead to legal action.
- Families have 1 to 12 years after birth to initiate legal action, depending on the state they live in.
- Nurses may be named in lawsuits.
- Nurses must remain competent in their field. *Nursing competence* is the ability to safely perform functions that demonstrate essential knowledge and skills that comply with the standard of care.
- Critical nursing skills include analyzing and interpreting fetal heart rate (FHR) tracings and uterine contraction patterns; acting in response to the physiology of fetal heart patterns and responding to/intervening in issues causing abnormal FHR tracings and uterine contraction patterns; acting to prevent injury to the patient and the fetus; advocating for and promoting the safety of the patient and the fetus; appropriately implementing and updating the plan of care and ensuring that the patient understands the plan of care; determining a nursing diagnosis and implementing a plan of care and interventions based on the nursing diagnosis; determining the physiologic meaning and implications of the FHR and uterine contraction patterns; and identifying and treating potential risks to the patient and the fetus.
- *Standard of care* is defined as the behavior of an ordinary, careful, reasonable, or prudent nurse. This includes investigating reasons for abnormal FHR patterns by obtaining all necessary data and implementing appropriate and timely interventions. Thus, an important standard of care is the competent and safe analysis of FHR patterns and uterine contraction patterns.
- *Substandard intrapartal care* is defined as a provider failing to give care that meets the appropriate standards of care.
- Sources of information that contribute to the determination of the standard of care include collaborative agreements; hospital bylaws, rules, and regulations; institutional policies, procedures, and protocols; publications, such as textbooks, journals, committee opinions, and practice bulletins; state licensure practice acts or rules and regulations; and professional organizations that create guidelines in the obstetrics and neonatal settings.
- Nurses must advocate for those who are not able to advocate for themselves due to fear, lack of knowledge, or inability.
- *Negligence* includes the concepts of duty, breach of duty, causation, and damages. *Duty* is to optimize outcomes and prevent injury. *Breach of duty* is the failure to meet the standard of care, which prevents fulfillment of the duty to prevent injury. *Causation* is the direct connection between the failure to meet the standard of care and the injury. *Damages* can result in monetary compensation for the patient. ►

Overview (*continued*)

- The chain of command should be written in institutional protocol. *Chain of command* reflects the organizational chart from the staff nurse to the chief nursing and medical officers. Some reasons for using the chain of command: Provider does not respond to calls or pages. Provider shows signs of impairment. Provider's actions will potentially cause patient endangerment. Provider exhibits behavior that is unprofessional or threatening.

Nursing Interventions

- Use the chain of command.
- Follow all institutional policies, procedures, and standards of care.
- Objectively document all actions and interactions and the time they occur and include specific details of what is being reported to the provider. *Example:* At 12:20 p.m., the nurse notified Dr. Jones of FHR of 60 bpm × 90 seconds with no response to interventions. The nurse requested Dr. Jones to the bedside for immediate evaluation of the FHR tracing. At 12:25 p.m., the nurse paged Dr. Jones for FHR of 60 bpm × 390 seconds, with no response from Dr. Jones. The nurse then called Dr. Smith for immediate evaluation of FHR tracing.

 **POP QUIZ 6.3**

A nurse is caring for a patient with a category III FHR tracing. The nurse calls the provider and leaves a message, but the provider does not respond. What is a priority for the nurse?

 **POP QUIZ 6.4**

A nurse is caring for a patient with a category III FHR tracing. The nurse calls the provider. The provider does not respond to numerous attempts to call, but the nurse continues to call the provider and does not use the chain of command and call the next person in charge. What is the legal implication for the nurse?

PATIENT SAFETY

Overview

- *Debriefing* is an important part of all patient safety events. Debriefing is confidential and uses a nonjudgmental approach. Debriefing should be done immediately (or as soon as possible) after the safety event; all team members involved should debrief to discuss what went well and what could be improved as a team. Debriefing is also used to provide support to other team members. There is no finger pointing or singling out of team members during debriefing.
- Patient safety is an essential component of commitment to the provision of optimal healthcare.
- A *patient safety event* is any event or action that leads to, or has the potential to lead to, a worsened patient outcome related to the event or action. Events may be related to systems, operations, drug administration, or any clinical aspect of patient care.
- Communication is an essential component of patient safety. Accurate, clear communication contributes to patient safety. The healthcare team may use a variety of communication tools and techniques to facilitate accurate, clear, and concise communication.
- Important steps to improve patient safety: Continuously review FHR tracings to maintain competence. Implement recommended safe medication practices. Improve communication among healthcare providers. Improve communication with patients and family members. Make safety a priority in every aspect of practice. Practice for emergencies by performing simulations. Recognize patients as full partners in care. Reduce the likelihood of surgical errors by using a surgery checklist, ensuring a time out has been called, and ensuring that the surgical site has been marked. Use teamwork and collaboration in the care of a patient. ▶

Overview (*continued*)

- *Just culture* holds organizations accountable for the systems they have designed. In addition, just culture holds the organization accountable for responding to the behaviors of its employees in a manner that is both fair and just: Adopt and develop safe practices that reduce the likelihood of system failures that can cause adverse outcomes. Most medication errors can be linked to a system failure—for example, care that is out of the nurse-to-patient ratio. Ensure that instances of adverse outcomes or failure to follow safety protocols are investigated fairly and openly. Ensure that nurses feel empowered to speak up when they are uncomfortable with an FHR tracing. Identify and study the patterns and causes of error occurrence within delivery. Identify FHR tracings that are not interpreted correctly. It is acceptable for the nurse to ask others to review an FHR tracing when uncertain of what is occurring.
- Just culture recognizes that some human error is inevitable.
- Just culture requires that nurses and providers recognize that the potential for errors exists.
- Just culture requires a learning environment that encourages disclosure and exchange of information in the event of errors, near misses, and adverse outcomes.
- Just culture recognizes the responsibility of all healthcare providers to follow safe practices and to avoid at-risk behaviors.
- Simulations are essential to enhance team skills in the obstetric (OB) setting. Simulations should include all multidisciplinary team members. Simulations should occur in a safe environment for learning and practice. Simulations improve the safety of the patient, fetus, and newborn, as well as enhance teamwork and communication among the healthcare team. Simulations promote interprofessional education and collaboration. Debriefing after simulation enhances team performance and improves clinician behavior and technical skills, as well as clinical performance and overall patient care. Simulations should offer opportunities for staff to ask questions and seek clarification as needed.

Nursing Interventions

- Communicate accurately and clearly using recognized tools and techniques.
- Debrief after each event.
- Report all patient safety events.
- Use the chain of command.

QUALITY IMPROVEMENT

Overview

- Quality improvement (QI) is a framework used to help improve healthcare and care of the patient.
- Concepts of QI include establishing a culture of quality in your area; determining and prioritizing potential areas for improvement; collecting and analyzing data; communicating results; committing to ongoing evaluation; and spreading successes by sharing lessons learned with others.
- Determine what needs improvement by collecting and using benchmark data. Some examples include breastfeeding rates, catheter-associated urinary tract infection rates, falls, neonatal birth traumas, and nulliparous term singleton vertex cesarean section rates. ►

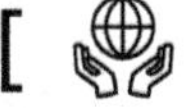

NURSING PEARL

Patient safety measures should be ongoing. All nurses and providers should use safe practices and encourage others to do so.

POP QUIZ 6.5

After a neonatal code in the operating room, team members discuss what went well and what could be improved. What is this an example of?

Overview (*continued*)

- Ensure QI: Implement evidence-based guidelines, improve outcomes, and use standardization within QI to decrease deviation in results.
- Use these best practices when implementing QI projects: Place a priority on encouraging communication, engagement, and participation for all of the stakeholders affected by the QI process. Start with a small multidisciplinary team that is vested. Start with small-scale changes. Use a standardized process, such as the PDSA (plan, do, study, act) cycle, to implement QI projects or measures.

Nursing Interventions

- Follow evidence-based guidelines.
- Implement a QI project and monitor clinical activity through observation and collection of data.
- Use standardization when possible.
- Include stakeholders in the process.
- Report the effects of changes that were implemented.
- Track progress of the implementation process.

[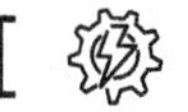] **ALERT!**

It is important to note that hospital payments from insurance companies may be based on outcomes from quality data.

[] **POP QUIZ 6.6**

What is the name of the process that can be used when implementing a QI project?

RESOURCES

Agency for Healthcare Research and Quality. (2017). *CUS tool—Improving communication and teamwork in the surgical environment module.* https://www.ahrq.gov/hai/tools/ambulatory-surgery/sections/implementation/training-tools/cus-tool.html

Agency for Healthcare Research and Quality. (2020). *Section 4: Ways to approach the quality improvement process.* https://www.ahrq.gov/cahps/quality-improvement/improvement-guide/4-approach-qi-process/index.html

American Academy of Family Physicians. (n.d). *Basics of quality improvement.* https://www.aafp.org/family-physician/practice-and-career/managing-your-practice/quality-improvement-basics.html

American College of Obstetricians and Gynecologists. (2007, Reaffirmed 2016). ACOG Committee Opinion No. 390: Ethical decision making in obstetrics and gynecology. *Obstetrics & Gynecology, 110*(6), 1479–1487. https://doi.org/10.1097/01.aog.0000291573.09193.36

American College of Obstetricians and Gynecologists. (2009). ACOG Committee Opinion No. 447: Patient safety in obstetrics and gynecology. *Obstetrics & Gynecology, 114*(6), 1424–1427. https://doi.org/10.1097/aog.0b013e3181c6f90e

Austin, N., Goldhaber-Fiebert, S., Daniels, K., Arafeh, J., Grenon, V., Welle, D., & Lipman, S. (2017). Building comprehensive strategies for obstetric safety: Simulation drills and communication. *Obstetric Anesthesia Digest, 37*(2), 61–62. https://doi.org/10.1097/01.aoa.0000515726.29190.ef

Birth Injury Help Center. (n.d.). *How long do you have to file a birth injury malpractice lawsuit?* https://www.birthinjuryhelpcenter.org/birth-injury-statute-of-limitations.html

Brigham and Women's Faulkner Hospital. (n.d.). *What is just culture? Changing the way we think about errors to improve patient safety and staff satisfaction.* https://www.brighamandwomensfaulkner.org/about-bwfh/news/what-is-just-culture-changing-the-way-we-think-about-errors-to-improve-patient-safety-and-staff-satisfaction

Centers for Medicare & Medicaid Services. (2021, December 1). *Quality measurement and quality improvement.* https://www.cms.gov/Medicare/Quality-Initiatives-Patient-Assessment-Instruments/MMS/Quality-Measure-and-Quality-Improvement-

Cheng, A., Grant, V., Dieckmann, P., Arora, S., Robinson, T., & Eppich, W. (2015). Faculty development for simulation programs: Five issues for the future of debriefing training. *Simulation in Healthcare: The Journal of the Society for Simulation in Healthcare, 10*(4), 217–222. https://doi.org/10.1097/SIH.0000000000000090

Harder, N. (2018). The value of simulation in health care: The obvious, the tangential, and the obscure. *Clinical Simulation in Nursing, 15*, 73–74. https://doi.org/10.1016/j.ecns.2017.12.004

Lippke, S., Derksen, C., Keller, F. M., Kötting, L., Schmiedhofer, M., & Welp, A. (2021). Effectiveness of communication interventions in obstetrics—A systematic review. *International Journal of Environmental Research and Public Health, 18*(5), 2616. https://doi.org/10.3390/ijerph18052616

OPLN Law. (2020, April 7). *Substandard quality of care: What you need to know.* https://lawnj.net/information/substandard-care

Schnipper, J. L., Fitall, E., Hall, K. K., & Gale, B. (2021, March 10). *Approach to improving patient safety: Communication.* Agency for Healthcare Research and Quality. https://psnet.ahrq.gov/perspective/approach-improving-patient-safety-communication

TRACINGS ANALYSIS PRACTICE

PATIENT CASE STUDIES

Read the following case studies and use the fetal heart rate (FHR) tracings to answer the questions.

Case Study 7.1

A 21-year-old patient is being evaluated for the first time. Based on the patient's subjective report, it is suspected that the patient is at 39 weeks' gestation. The FHR tracing is shown in Figure 7.1. Interpret the tracing and determine the priority interventions, if any, for the nurse caring for this patient.

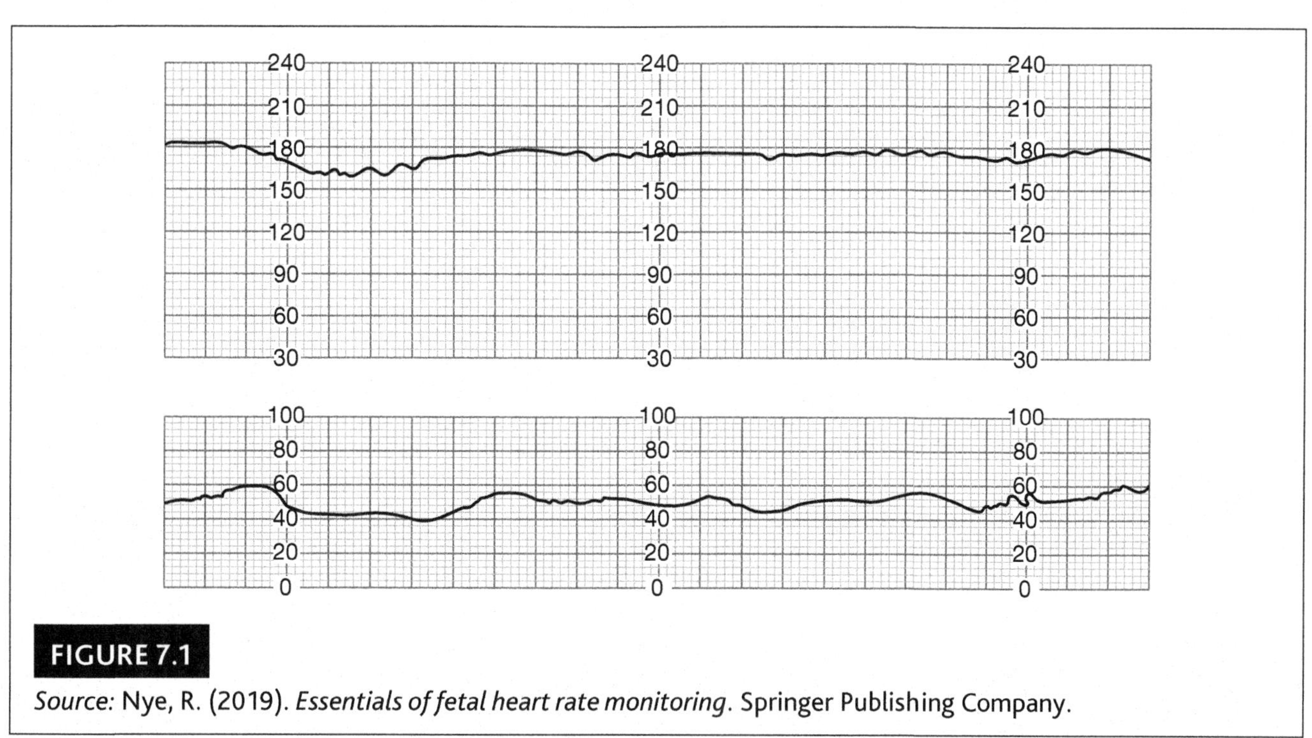

FIGURE 7.1

Source: Nye, R. (2019). *Essentials of fetal heart rate monitoring.* Springer Publishing Company.

Heart rate:
FHR category:
Variability:
Acceleration (Y/N):
Deceleration (Y/N):
Type of deceleration:

Answers
Heart rate: 180
FHR category: II
Variability: Minimal
Acceleration (Y/N): N
Deceleration (Y/N): Y
Type of deceleration: Late
The tracing shows the presence of tachycardia, minimal variability, and late decelerations, indicating that the fetus is oxygen deprived. The priority nursing interventions include the following:

- Notify the provider.
- Place an intravenous (IV) line.
- Start an IV fluid bolus infusion (normal saline or lactated Ringer's solution).
- Place patient on side.
- Administer oxygen.
- Prepare for emergent delivery.

Case Study 7.2

A 29-year-old patient is in labor. The patient's cervix measures 6 cm dilated. Butorphanol and promethazine were administered 30 minutes ago for pain relief. Interpret the FHR tracing shown in Figure 7.2 and determine the most appropriate nursing intervention, if any.

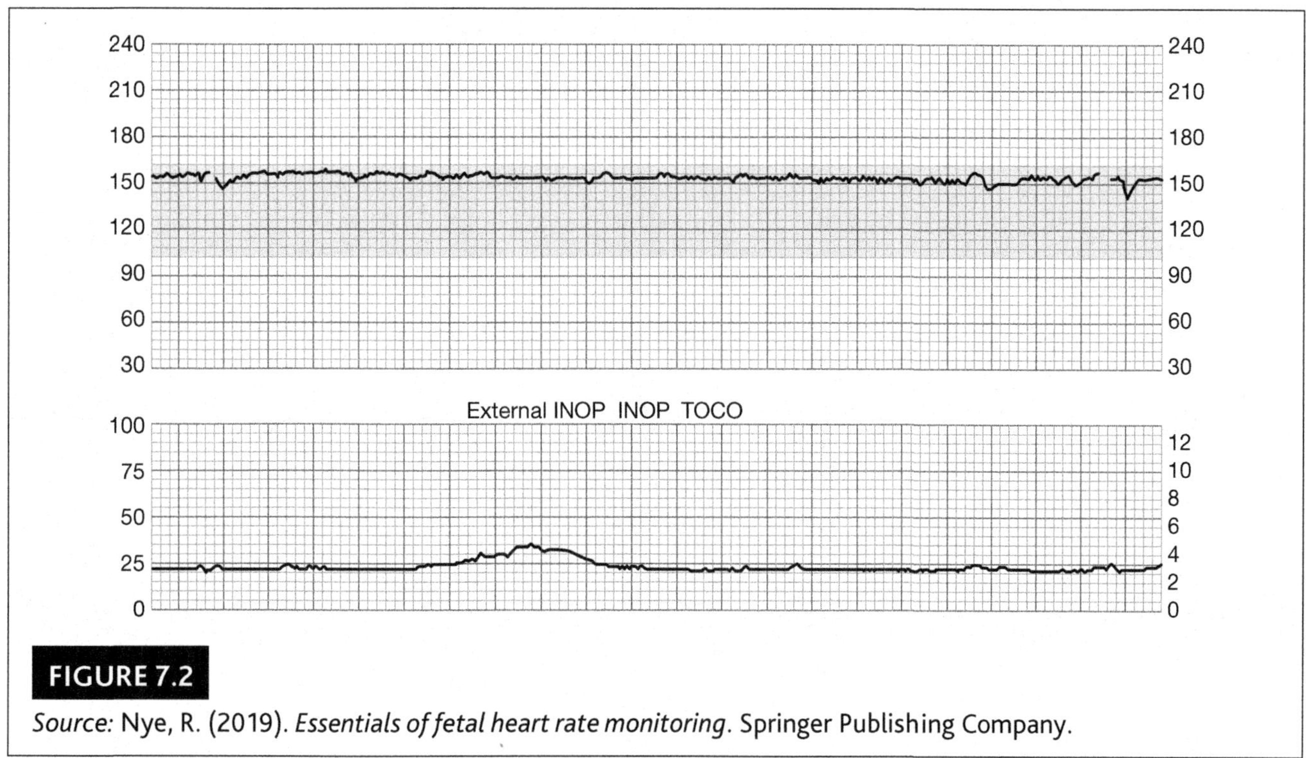

FIGURE 7.2

Source: Nye, R. (2019). *Essentials of fetal heart rate monitoring.* Springer Publishing Company.

Heart rate:
FHR category:
Variability:
Acceleration (Y/N):
Deceleration (Y/N):
Type of deceleration:

Answers
Heart rate: 150
FHR category: II
Variability: Minimal
Acceleration (Y/N): N
Deceleration (Y/N): N
Type of deceleration: None
No intervention is required. This is an expected finding after a patient has received butorphanol because narcotics can cause a decrease in the variability and frequency of accelerations.

Case Study 7.3

A 33-year-old patient at 40 weeks' and 2 days' gestation has been administered oxytocin for induction of labor. The FHR tracing is shown in Figure 7.3. Interpret the tracing and determine what, if any, nursing interventions are needed.

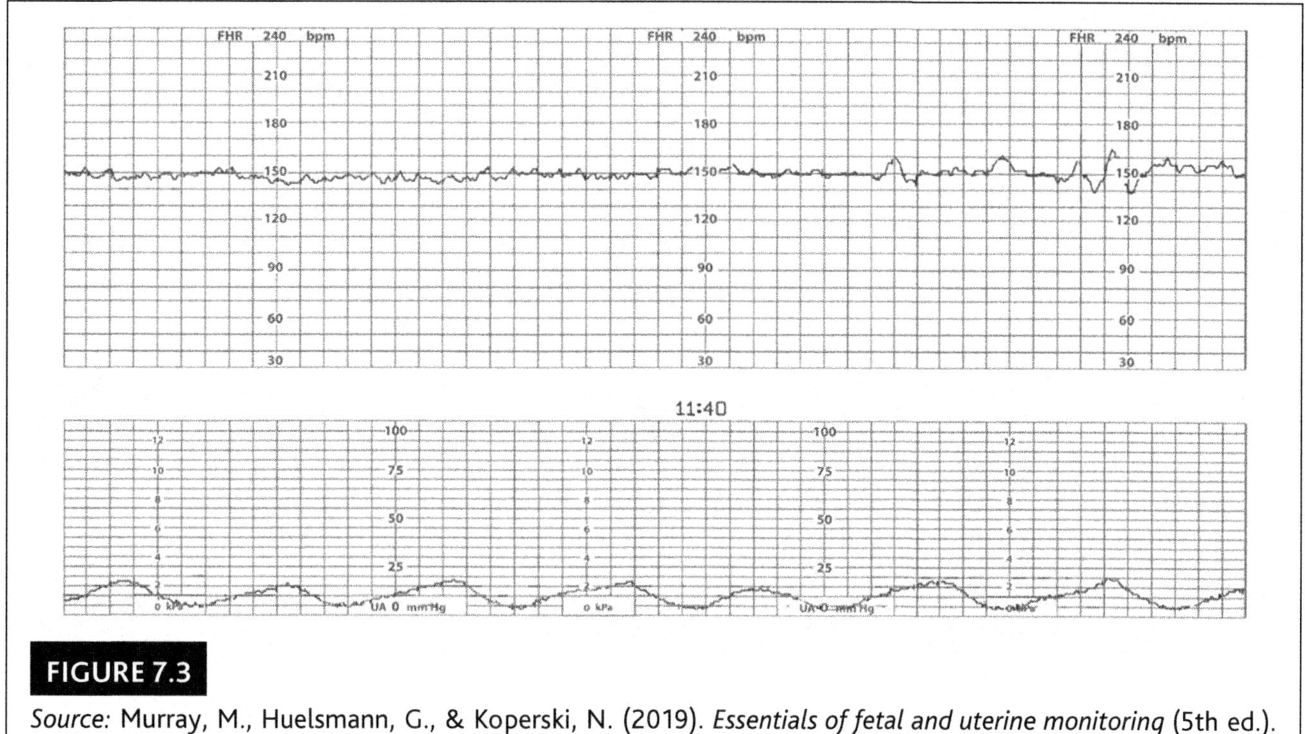

FIGURE 7.3

Source: Murray, M., Huelsmann, G., & Koperski, N. (2019). *Essentials of fetal and uterine monitoring* (5th ed.). Springer Publishing Company.

Heart rate:

FHR category:

Variability:

Acceleration (Y/N):

Deceleration (Y/N):

Type of deceleration:

Answers
Heart rate: 150
FHR category: II
Variability: Minimal
Acceleration (Y/N): N
Deceleration (Y/N): N
Type of deceleration: None
The tracing shows uterine tachysystole. The priority nursing interventions include the following:

- Discontinue the oxytocin.
- Reposition the patient.
- Administer an IV fluid bolus (normal saline or lactated Ringer's solution).

Case Study 7.4

A 24-year-old patient received an epidural 10 minutes ago. The FHR tracing is pictured in Figure 7.4. Interpret the tracing and describe the required nursing interventions, if any.

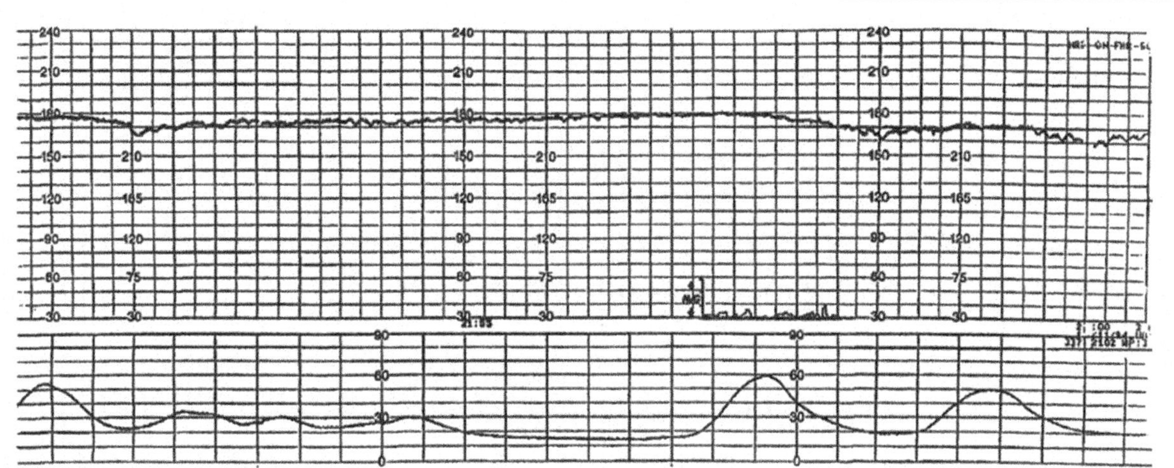

FIGURE 7.4

Source: Murray, M., Huelsmann, G., & Koperski, N. (2019). *Essentials of fetal and uterine monitoring* (5th ed.). Springer Publishing Company.

Heart rate:
FHR category:
Variability:
Acceleration (Y/N):
Deceleration (Y/N):
Type of deceleration:

Answers
Heart rate: 155
FHR category: II
Variability: Minimal
Acceleration (Y/N): N
Deceleration (Y/N): Y
Type of deceleration: Late
The tracing shows late decelerations, most likely caused by patient hypotension due to the epidural admin-istration. Nursing interventions include the following:

- Notify the provider.
- Place patient on side.
- Administer an IV fluid bolus (normal saline or lactated Ringer's solution).
- Administer oxygen.

Case Study 7.5

A 22-year-old full-term patient is placed on the monitor. It is the patient's first pregnancy. The FHR tracing is shown in Figure 7.5. Interpret the tracing, determine the patient's FHR, and describe what the interpretation indicates is occurring. List any nursing interventions that are required.

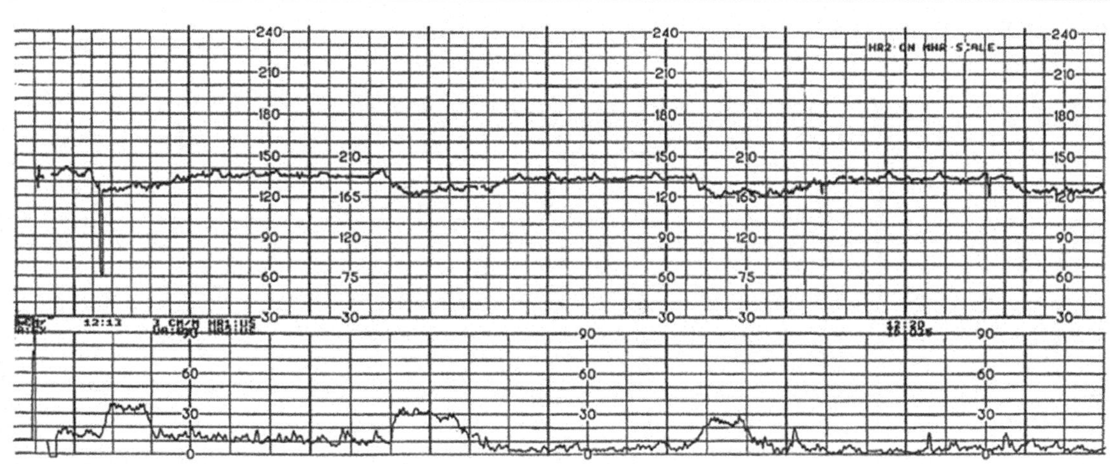

FIGURE 7.5

Source: Murray, M., Huelsmann, G., & Koperski, N. (2019). *Essentials of fetal and uterine monitoring* (5th ed.). Springer Publishing Company.

Heart rate:
FHR category:
Variability:
Acceleration (Y/N):
Deceleration (Y/N):
Type of deceleration:

Answers
Heart rate: 135
FHR category: I
Variability: Moderate
Acceleration (Y/N): N
Deceleration (Y/N): Y
Type of deceleration: Early
The tracing shows early decelerations, which are an expected finding indicating that labor is progressing. The nurse should continue to monitor the patient, but no other interventions are necessary at this time.

Case Study 7.6

A 19-year-old patient of unknown gestation is being evaluated for abdominal pain and to rule out contractions. The patient has no history of previous prenatal care and shows signs of substance use. Interpret the patient's FHR tracing in Figure 7.6, describe the likely cause, and indicate the priority nursing interventions, if any.

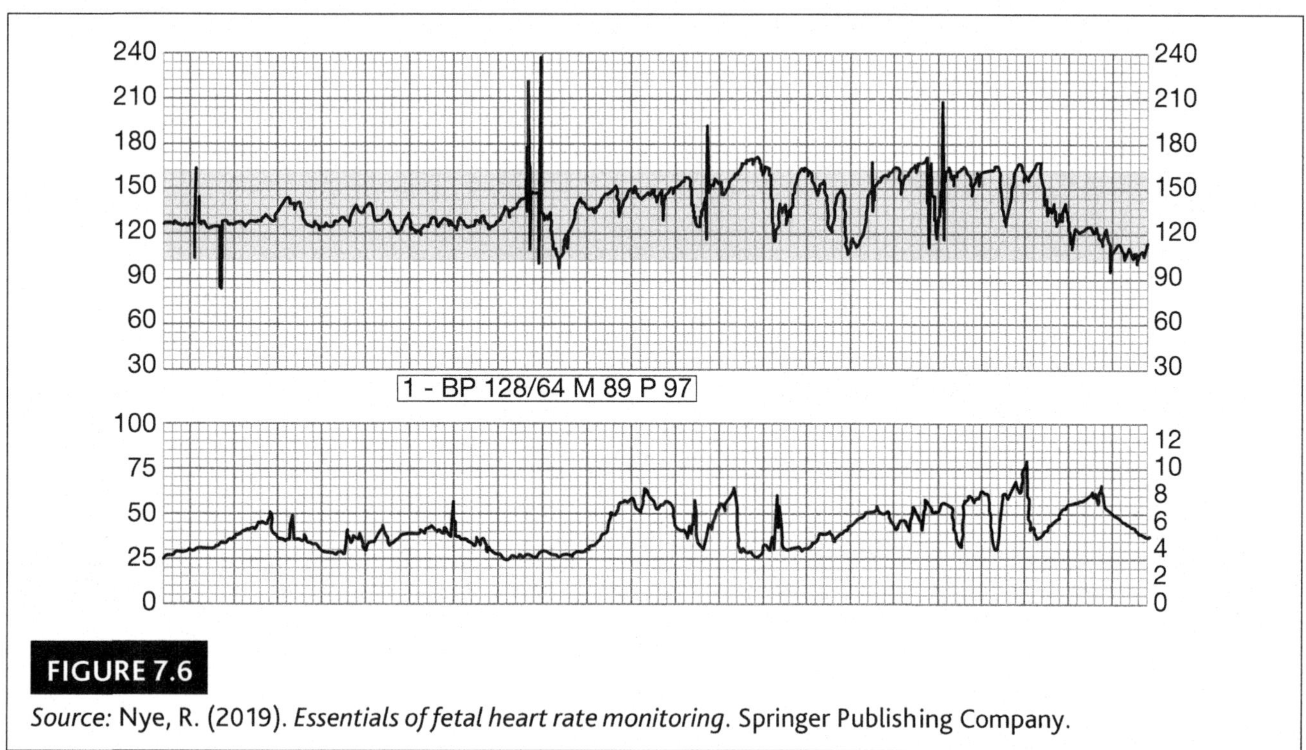

FIGURE 7.6

Source: Nye, R. (2019). *Essentials of fetal heart rate monitoring.* Springer Publishing Company.

Heart rate:

FHR category:

Variability:

Acceleration (Y/N):

Deceleration (Y/N):

Type of deceleration:

Answers
Heart rate: 125
FHR category: II
Variability: Marked
Acceleration (Y/N): Y
Deceleration (Y/N): N
Type of deceleration: None
The FHR tracing may indicate substance use. The priority nursing actions are to initiate monitoring of the patient and the fetus and to notify the provider.

Case Study 7.7

A 32-year-old patient who is 39 weeks' and 6 days' gestation presents in labor and requests an epidural. Interpret the patient's FHR tracing in Figure 7.7 and determine whether the fetus is acidotic. What nursing interventions, if any, are required?

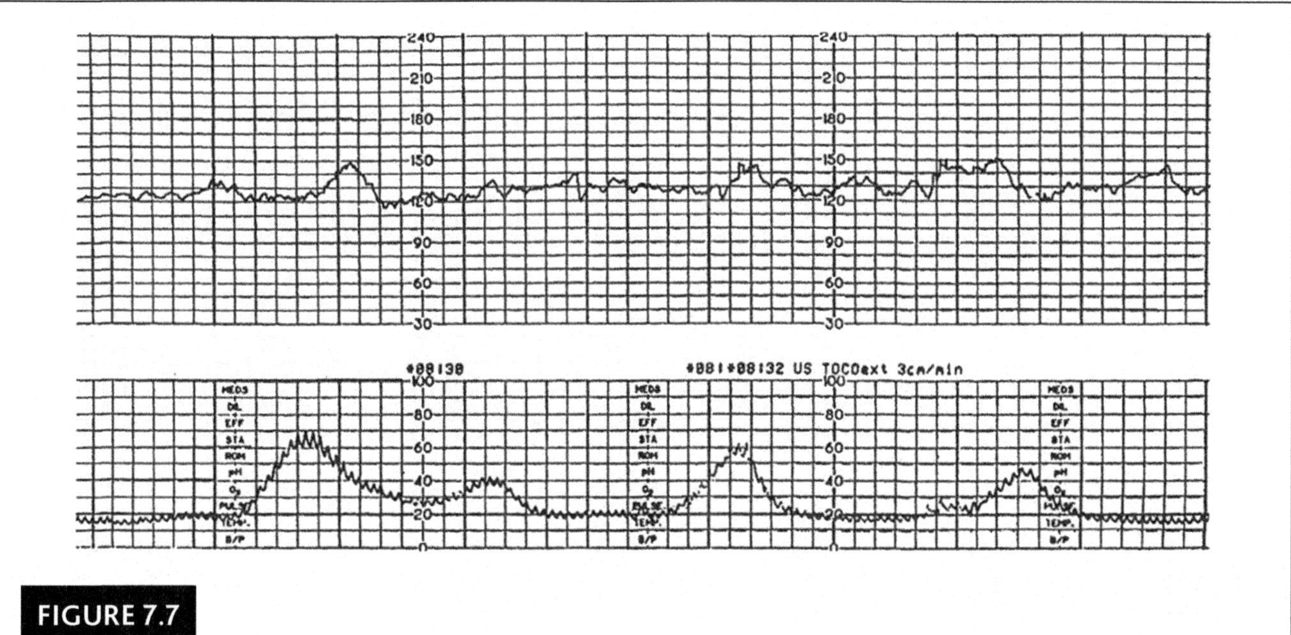

FIGURE 7.7

Source: Murray, M., Huelsmann, G., & Koperski, N. (2019). *Essentials of fetal and uterine monitoring* (5th ed.). Springer Publishing Company.

Heart rate:

FHR category:

Variability:

Acceleration (Y/N):

Deceleration (Y/N):

Type of deceleration:

Answers

Heart rate: 130
FHR category: I
Variability: Moderate
Acceleration (Y/N): Y
Deceleration (Y/N): N
Type of deceleration: None
This is a category I FHR tracing with a normal baseline, moderate variability, and accelerations present, indicating a nonacidotic fetus. No nursing interventions are currently required, but the nurse should continue to monitor per protocol.

Case Study 7.8

A patient received oxytocin to augment labor. Interpret the patient's FHR tracing in Figure 7.8 and indicate any required nursing interventions.

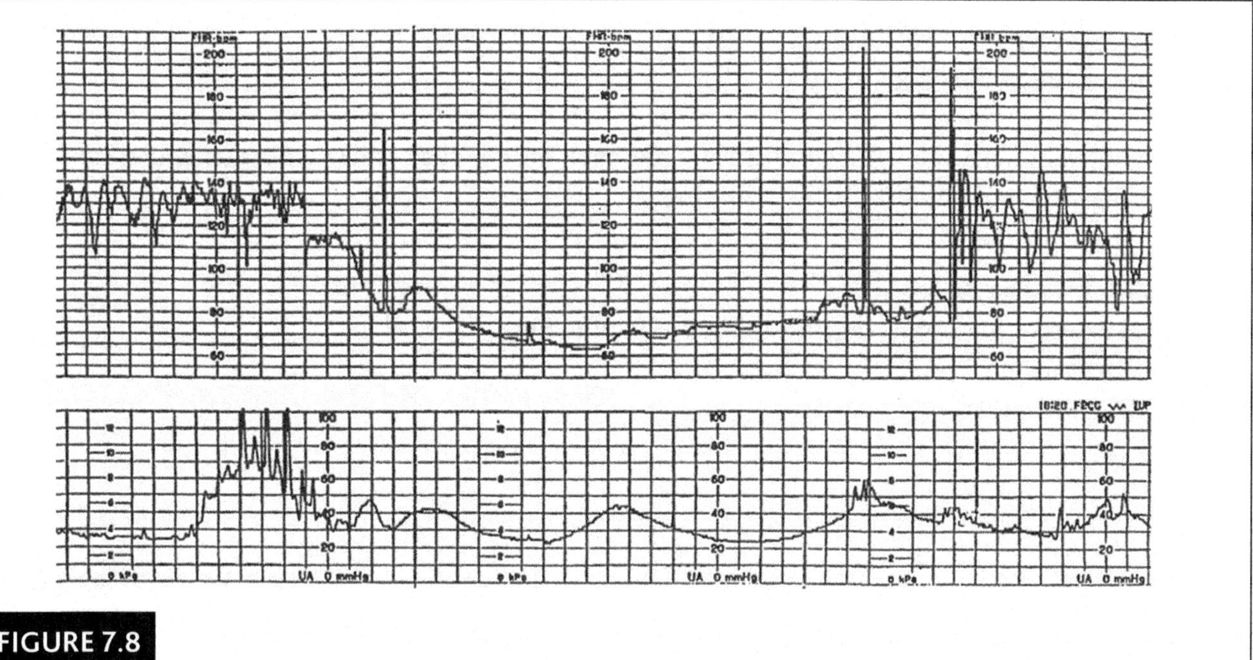

FIGURE 7.8

Source: Murray, M., Huelsmann, G., & Koperski, N. (2019). *Essentials of fetal and uterine monitoring* (5th ed.). Springer Publishing Company.

Heart rate:

FHR category:

Variability:

Acceleration (Y/N):

Deceleration (Y/N):

Type of deceleration:

Answers
Heart rate: Indeterminate
FHR category: II
Variability: Marked
Acceleration (Y/N): N
Deceleration (Y/N): Y
Type of deceleration: Prolonged
The FHR reveals a prolonged deceleration. The deceleration is classified as prolonged because it lasts longer than 2 minutes but less than 10 minutes. The prolonged deceleration is likely caused by uterine tachysystole. Nursing interventions include the following:

- Notify the provider.
- Discontinue the oxytocin.
- Administer an IV fluid bolus (normal saline or lactated Ringer's solution).
- Administer oxygen.
- Reposition the patient.

Case Study 7.9

A patient is being induced with oxytocin at 40 weeks' and 4 days' gestation. Interpret the patient's FHR tracing (Figure 7.9) and identify the area of greatest concern.

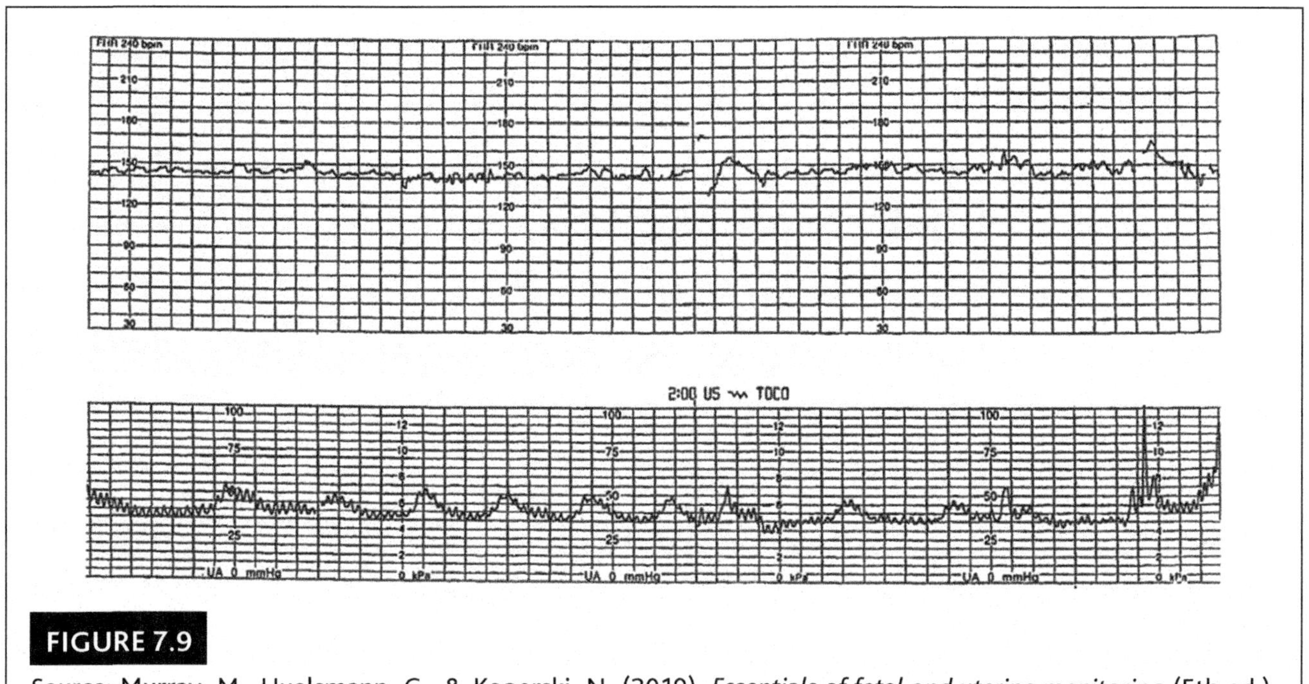

FIGURE 7.9

Source: Murray, M., Huelsmann, G., & Koperski, N. (2019). *Essentials of fetal and uterine monitoring* (5th ed.). Springer Publishing Company.

Heart rate:

FHR category:

Variability:

Acceleration (Y/N):

Deceleration (Y/N):

Type of deceleration:

Answers
Heart rate: 145
FHR category: I
Variability: Moderate
Acceleration (Y/N): Y
Deceleration (Y/N): N
Type of deceleration: None
The FHR tracing indicates uterine tachysystole, which leads to decreased fetal oxygenation and must be corrected. The nurse should discontinue the oxytocin, administer an IV fluid bolus (normal saline or lactated Ringer's solution), and notify the provider.

Case Study 7.10

A patient in labor receives an epidural. The FHR tracing in Figure 7.10 is obtained 10 minutes later. Interpret the tracing and identify any priority nursing interventions.

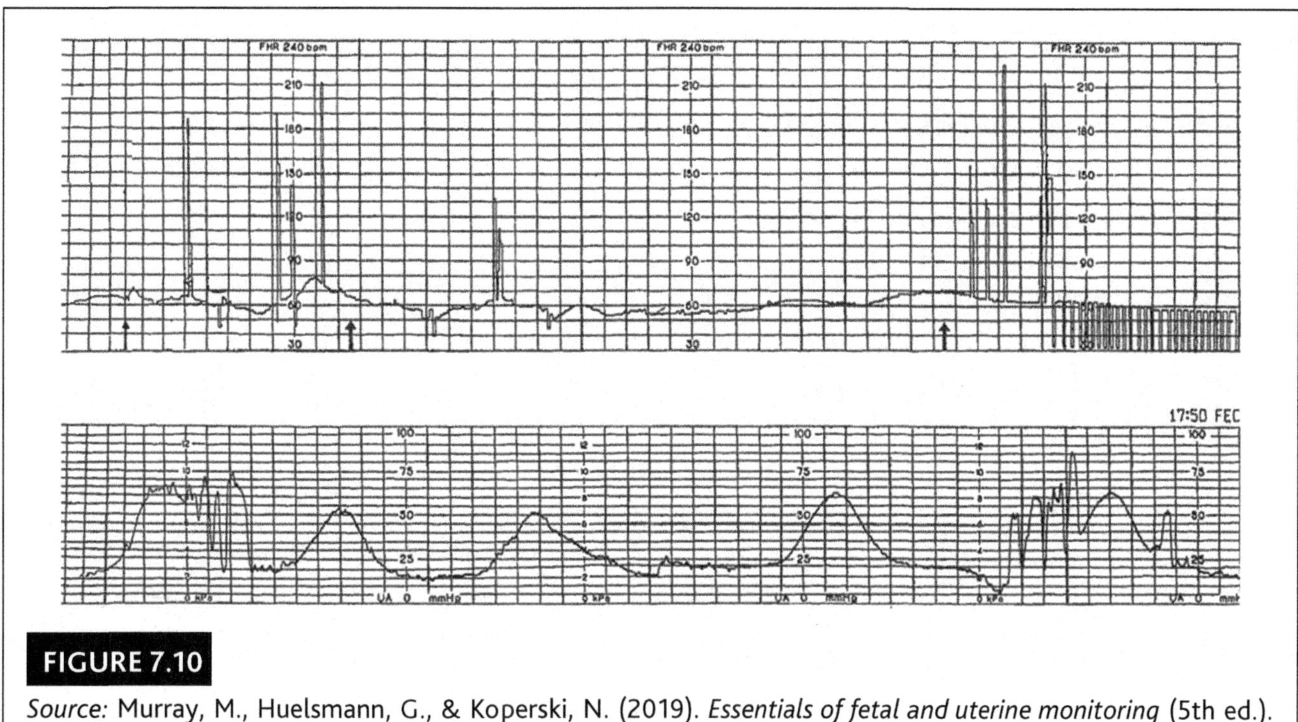

FIGURE 7.10

Source: Murray, M., Huelsmann, G., & Koperski, N. (2019). *Essentials of fetal and uterine monitoring* (5th ed.). Springer Publishing Company.

Heart rate:

FHR category:

Variability:

Acceleration (Y/N):

Deceleration (Y/N):

Type of deceleration:

Answers
Heart rate: 60 (bradycardia)
FHR category: III
Variability: Minimal
Acceleration (Y/N): Y
Deceleration (Y/N): N
Type of deceleration: None
This FHR tracing indicates fetal bradycardia, most likely due to maternal hypotension after epidural anesthesia. The nurse should do the following:

- Call the provider to the bedside immediately.
- Discontinue oxytocin.
- Administer oxygen.
- Administer an IV fluid bolus (normal saline or lactated Ringer's solution).
- Reposition the patient.

Case Study 7.11

A 17-year-old patient arrives via ambulance with severe abdominal pain and vaginal bleeding. The patient is at 32 weeks' gestation and has a history of substance use. What category is the FHR tracing (Figure 7.11), and what is the likely cause? What nursing interventions, if any, are necessary?

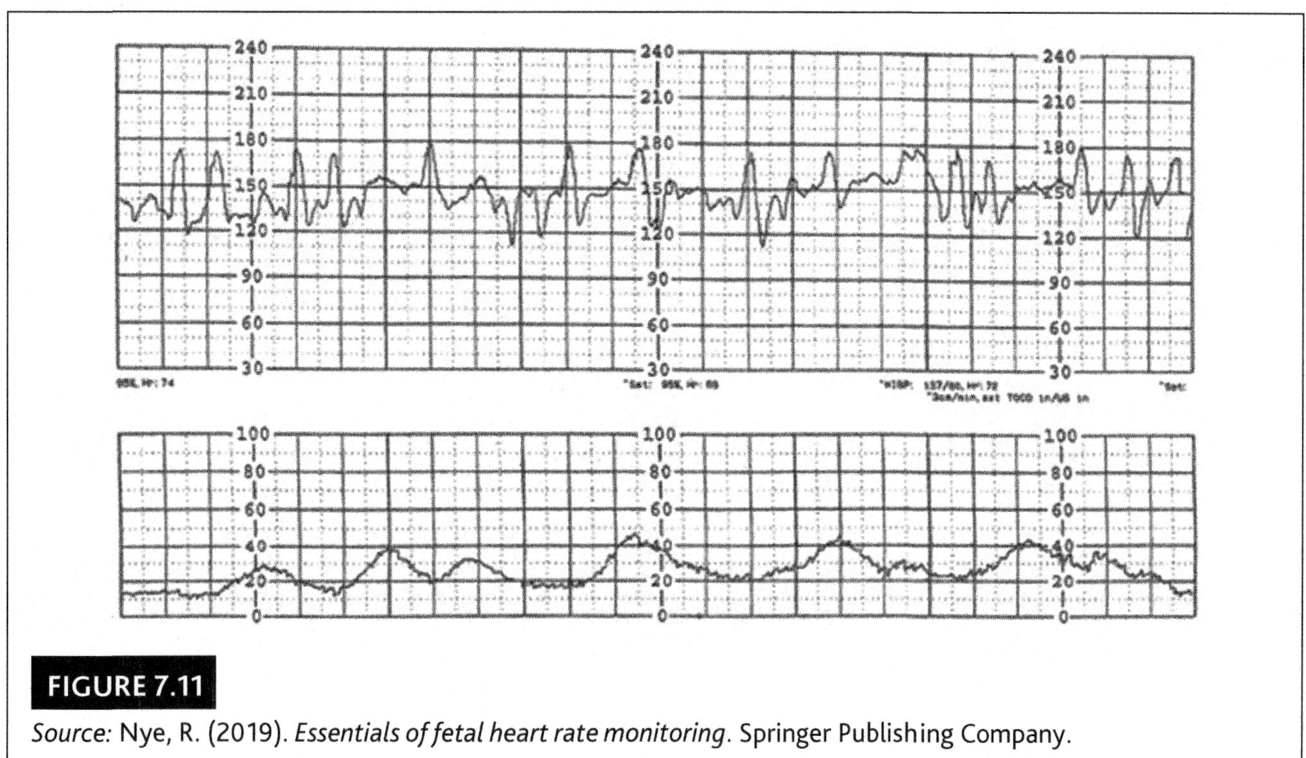

FIGURE 7.11

Source: Nye, R. (2019). *Essentials of fetal heart rate monitoring.* Springer Publishing Company.

Heart rate:

FHR category:

Variability:

Acceleration (Y/N):

Deceleration (Y/N):

Type of deceleration:

Answers
Heart rate: Indeterminate
FHR category: II
Variability: Marked
Acceleration (Y/N): N
Deceleration (Y/N): N
Type of deceleration: None
Because of the history of substance use; the painful, rigid abdomen; and the frequent contractions, the most likely cause is a placental abruption. Nursing interventions include placing the patient on their side, administering an IV fluid bolus (normal saline or lactated Ringer's solution), administering oxygen, notifying the provider, and preparing for emergent delivery.

Case Study 7.12

A 24-year-old patient at 41 weeks' gestation is being evaluated for reported decreased fetal movement since waking up this morning. Interpret the FHR tracing in Figure 7.12 and identify the priority nursing interventions, if any.

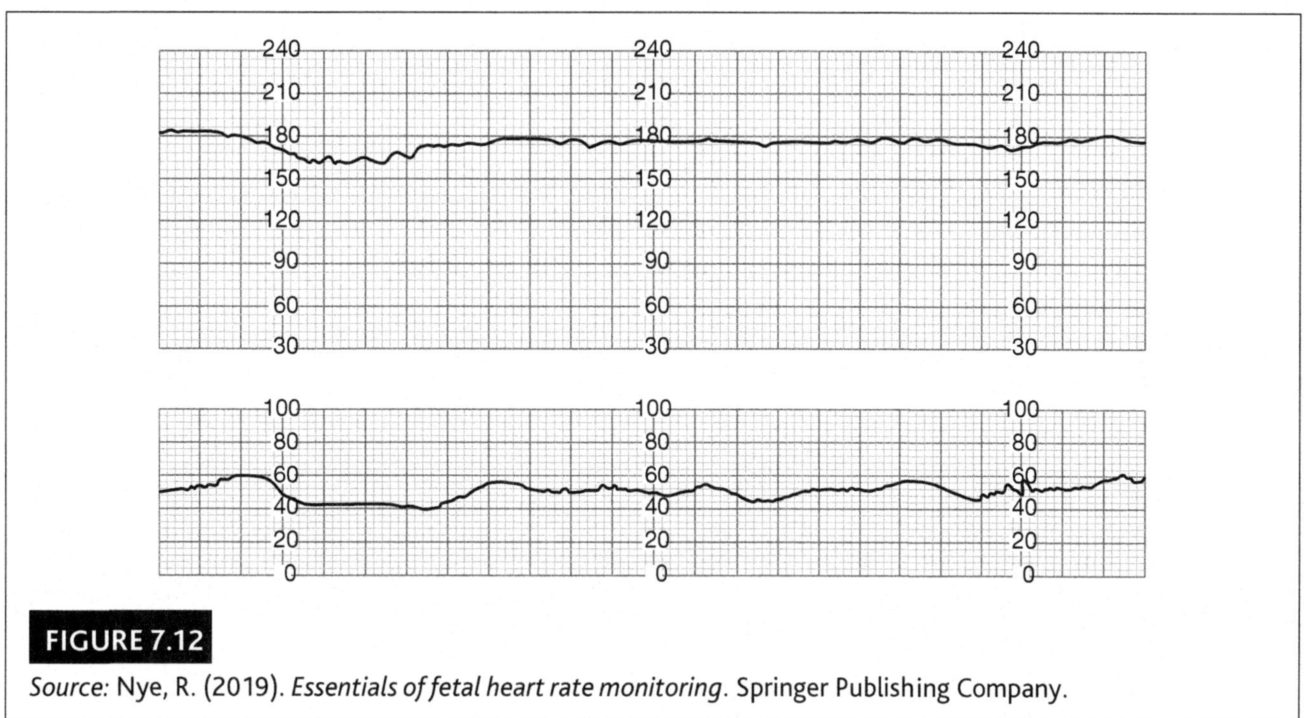

FIGURE 7.12

Source: Nye, R. (2019). *Essentials of fetal heart rate monitoring.* Springer Publishing Company.

Heart rate:
FHR category:
Variability:
Acceleration (Y/N):
Deceleration (Y/N):
Type of deceleration:

Answers
Heart rate: 180
FHR category: II
Variability: Minimal
Acceleration (Y/N): N
Deceleration (Y/N): Y
Type of deceleration: Late
The FHR tracing confirms decreased fetal movement, which indicates that the fetus is being deprived of oxygen. The nurse's priority interventions include the following:

- Notify the provider.
- Activate the emergency call system for other healthcare team members to provide immediate assistance.
- Administer an IV fluid bolus (normal saline or lactated Ringer's solution).
- Place patient on side.
- Administer oxygen.
- Prepare for emergent delivery.

Case Study 7.13

A patient presents for induction of labor at 41 weeks' and 2 days' gestation. It is the patient's first pregnancy. The cervical examination is 2 cm/30%/–3. The provider orders a cervical ripening agent. Interpret the FHR tracing in Figure 7.13 and indicate the next step for the nurse.

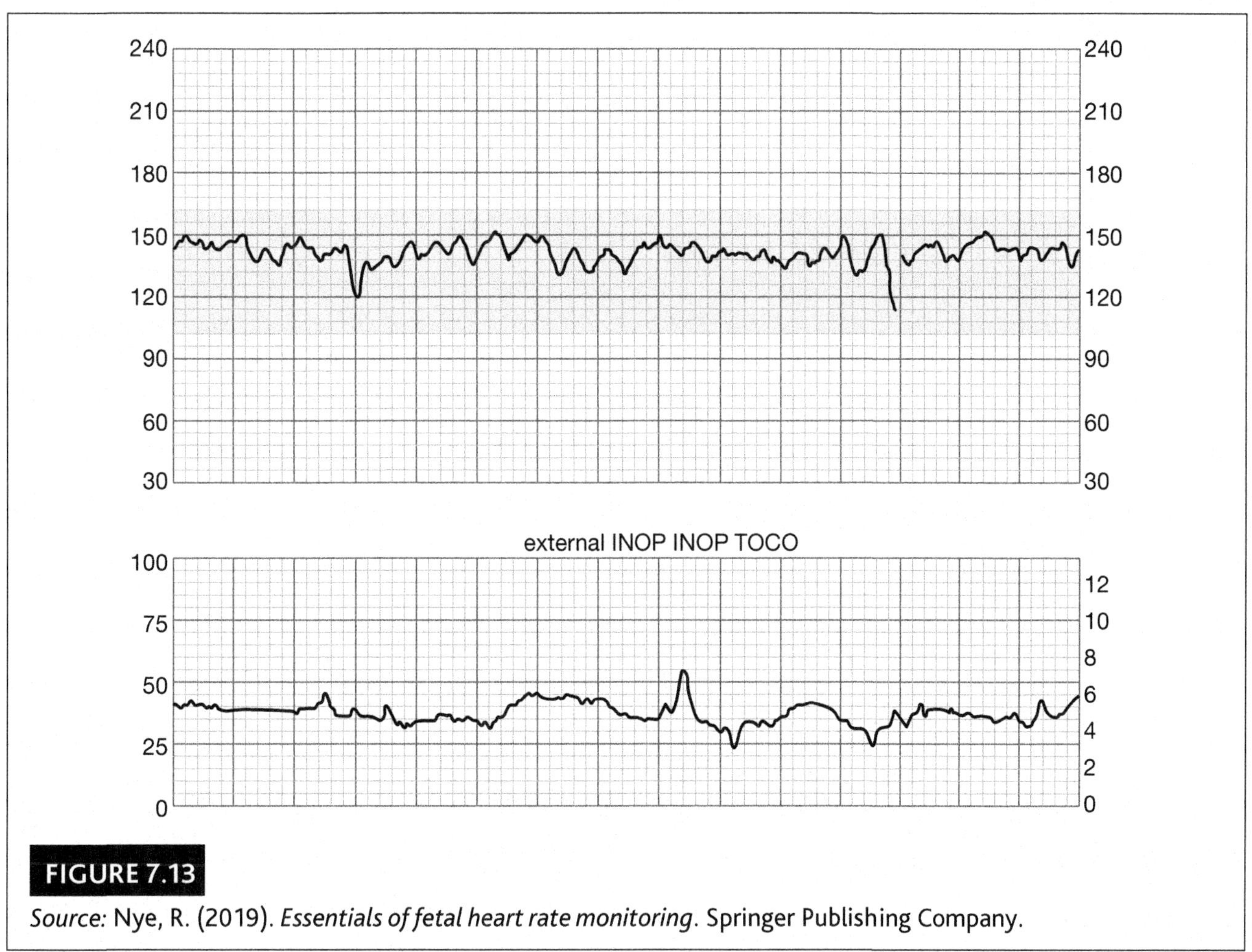

FIGURE 7.13

Source: Nye, R. (2019). *Essentials of fetal heart rate monitoring.* Springer Publishing Company.

Heart rate:
FHR category:
Variability:
Acceleration (Y/N):
Deceleration (Y/N):
Type of deceleration:

Answers
Heart rate: 140
FHR category: I
Variability: Moderate
Acceleration (Y/N): N
Deceleration (Y/N): N
Type of deceleration: None
The FHR is category I. The next step for the nurse is to administer the cervical ripening agent as ordered.

Case Study 7.14

A patient has had ruptured membranes for 32 hours. The patient was induced with oxytocin and is now dilated to 10 cm and is pushing. Interpret the patient's FHR tracing (Figure 7.14), and indicate the likely cause of the findings. What nursing interventions, if any, are required?

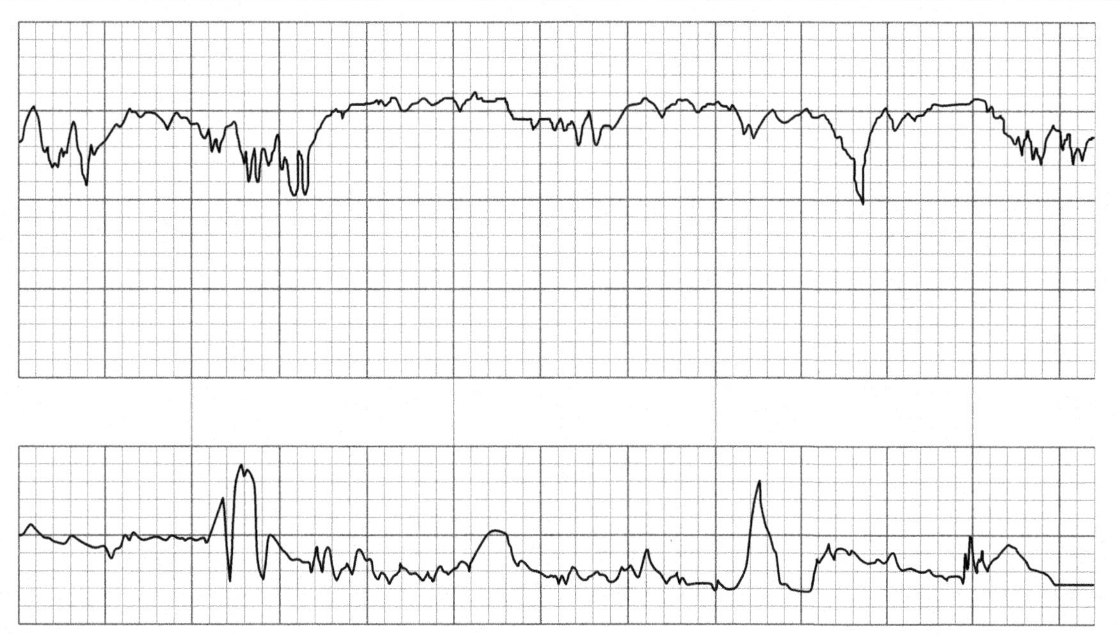

FIGURE 7.14

Source: National Certification Corporation. (2021). *Fetal assessment and safe labor management* (Appendix A). https://www.nccwebsite.org/content/documents/cms/2016_ncc_monograph_free_version.pdf. (NCC does not sponsor or endorse this resource, nor does it have a proprietary relationship with Springer Publishing Company.)

Heart rate:
FHR category:
Variability:
Acceleration (Y/N):
Deceleration (Y/N):
Type of deceleration:

Answers
Heart rate: 180
FHR category: II
Variability: Moderate
Acceleration (Y/N): N
Deceleration (Y/N): Y
Type of deceleration: Late, variable
The patient may have chorioamnionitis. The nurse should:

- Monitor the patient's temperature.
- Reposition the patient.
- Administer an IV fluid bolus (normal saline or lactated Ringer's solution).
- Discontinue the oxytocin.
- Encourage the patient to push with every second or third contraction.

Case Study 7.15

A 30-year-old patient with preeclampsia is admitted for evaluation of new-onset headache and reported decreased fetal movement. Interpret the initial FHR tracing in Figure 7.15, and identify the priority nursing interventions, if any.

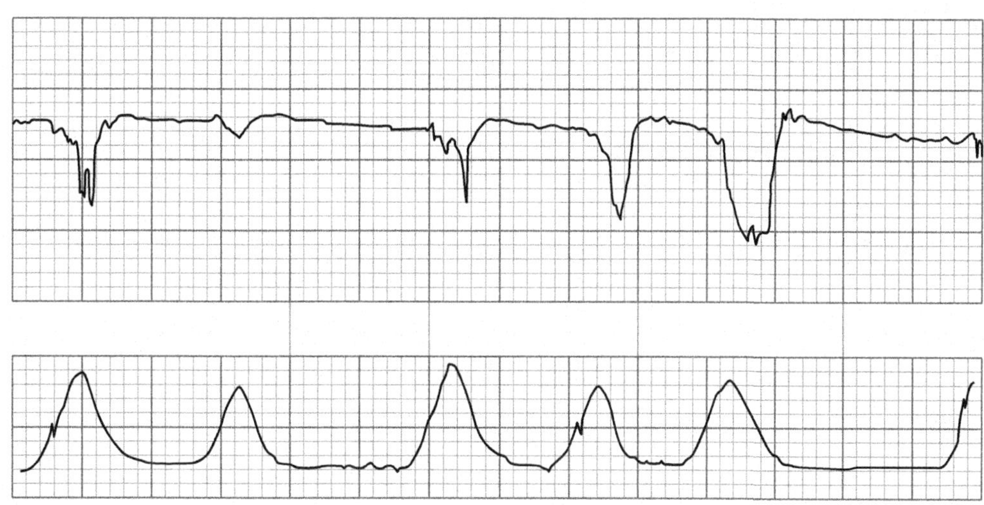

FIGURE 7.15

Source: National Certification Corporation. (2021). *Fetal assessment and safe labor management* (Appendix C). https://www.nccwebsite.org/content/documents/cms/2016_ncc_monograph_free_version.pdf. (NCC does not sponsor or endorse this resource, nor does it have a proprietary relationship with Springer Publishing Company.)

Heart rate:
FHR category:
Variability:
Acceleration (Y/N):
Deceleration (Y/N):
Type of deceleration:

Answers
Heart rate: 150
FHR category: III
Variability: Absent
Acceleration (Y/N): N
Deceleration (Y/N): Y
Type of deceleration: Variable
The FHR is a category III tracing that requires immediate intervention. Nursing interventions include the following:

- Call the provider.
- Start an IV.
- Administer an IV fluid bolus (normal saline or lactated Ringer's solution).
- Administer oxygen.
- Place patient on side.
- Prepare the patient for an emergency cesarean section.

Case Study 7.16

A patient is admitted for cervical ripening before induction. The provider sees the FHR and provides fetal scalp stimulation with a vaginal examination. What are some possible causes for the FHR shown in Figure 7.16, and what interventions are needed, if any?

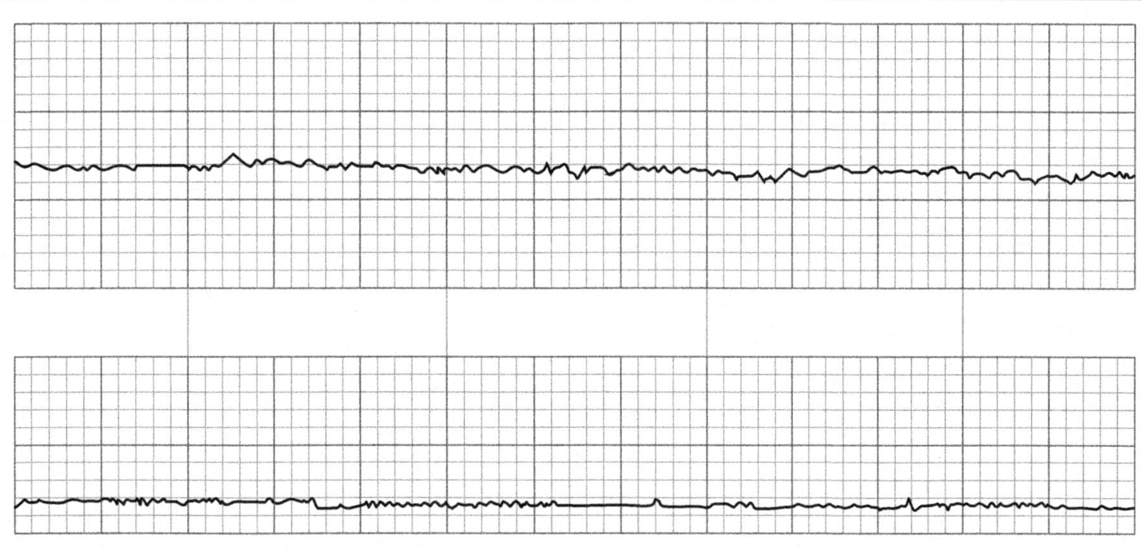

FIGURE 7.16

Source: National Certification Corporation. (2021). *Fetal assessment and safe labor management* (Appendix C). https://www.nccwebsite.org/content/documents/cms/2016_ncc_monograph_free_version.pdf. (NCC does not sponsor or endorse this resource, nor does it have a proprietary relationship with Springer Publishing Company.)

Heart rate:
FHR category:
Variability:
Acceleration (Y/N):
Deceleration (Y/N):
Type of deceleration:

Answers
Heart rate: 140
FHR category: II
Variability: Minimal
Acceleration (Y/N): N
Deceleration (Y/N): N
Type of deceleration: None
It is important to monitor the FHR and the patient because no acceleration after fetal scalp stimulation is an abnormal and concerning finding. While the fetus may be in a sleep cycle, possible concerning causes of no acceleration after fetal scalp stimulation include a neurologic or cardiac issue or hypoxia. Nursing interventions include the following:

- Call the provider.
- Start an IV.
- Administer an IV fluid bolus (normal saline or lactated Ringer's solution).
- Administer oxygen.
- Place patient on side.

Case Study 7.17

A 28-year-old patient with Sjögren syndrome is admitted in labor at 39 weeks. Interpret the FHR in Figure 7.17, identify the likely cause of the tracing, and list any necessary nursing interventions.

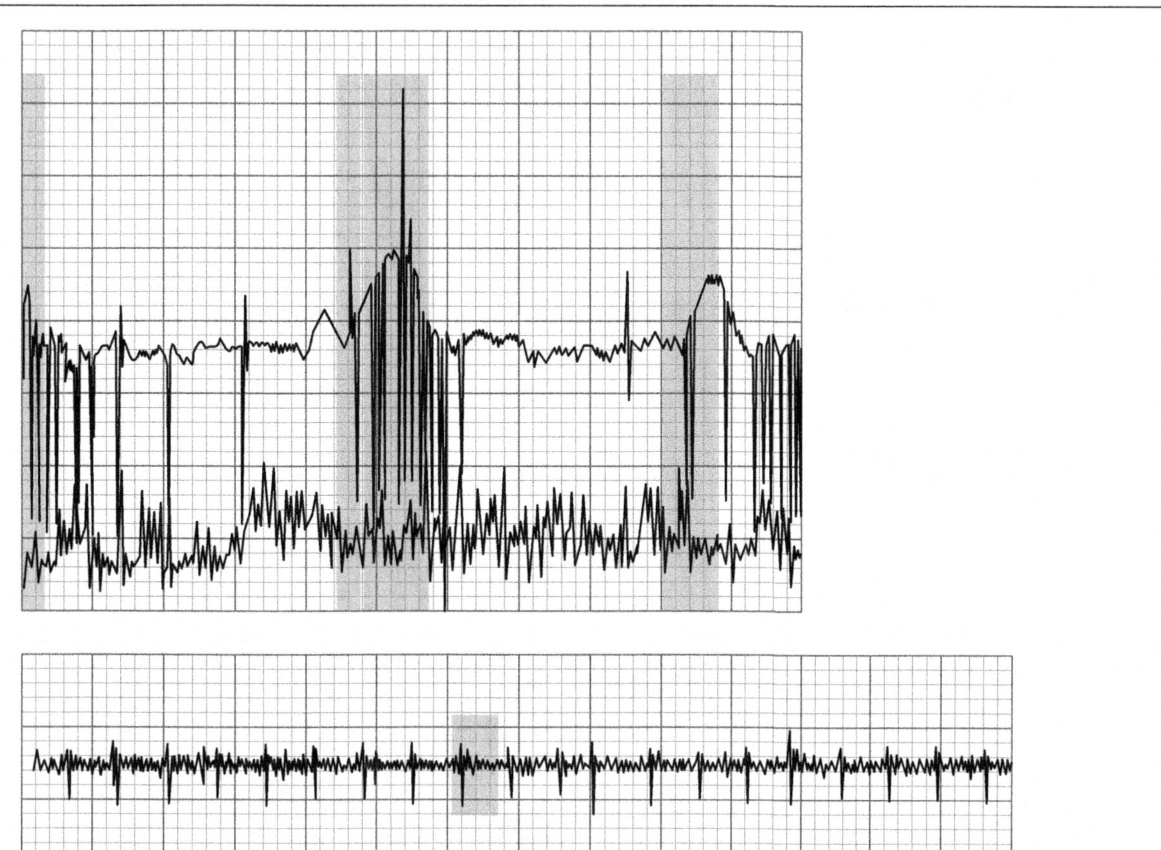

FIGURE 7.17

Source: Lakhno, I., Behar, J. A., Oster, J., Shulgin, V., Ostras, O., & Andreotti, F. (2017). The use of non-invasive fetal electrocardiography in diagnosing second-degree fetal atrioventricular block (Fig. 3). *Maternal Health, Neonatology and Perinatology, 3*, Article 14. https://doi.org/10.1186/s40748-017-0053-1

Heart rate:
FHR category:
Variability:
Acceleration (Y/N):
Deceleration (Y/N):
Type of deceleration:

Answers
Heart rate: 120
FHR category: I
Variability: Moderate
Acceleration (Y/N): Y
Deceleration (Y/N): N
Type of deceleration: None
The FHR is reactive but shows dropped beats. The most likely cause of this tracing is heart block owing to Sjögren syndrome. Nursing interventions include the following:

- Call the provider.
- Start an IV.
- Administer an IV fluid bolus (normal saline or lactated Ringer's solution).
- Administer oxygen.
- Place patient on side.

Case Study 7.18

A 20-year-old patient is 10 cm dilated and begins pushing. Interpret the patient's FHR tracing (Figure 7.18), and identify the most appropriate nursing interventions.

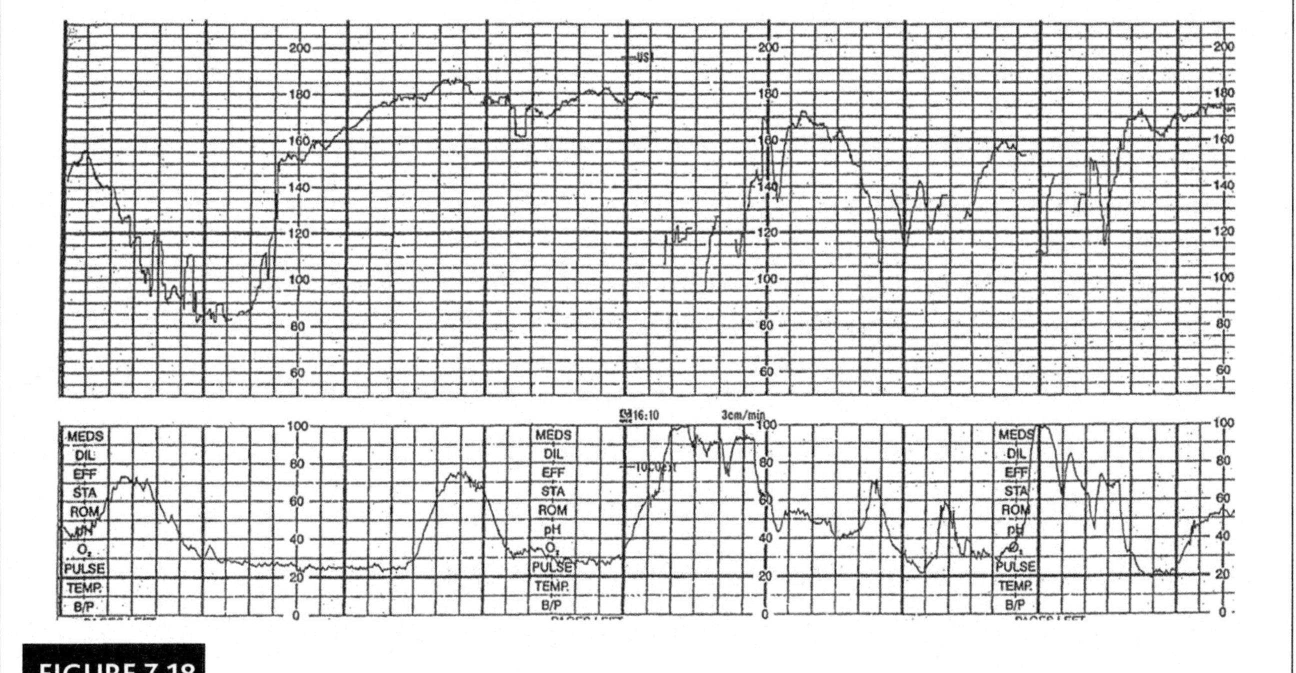

FIGURE 7.18

Source: Murray, M., Huelsmann, G., & Koperski, N. (2019). *Essentials of fetal and uterine monitoring* (5th ed.). Springer Publishing Company.

Heart rate:

FHR category:

Variability:

Acceleration (Y/N):

Deceleration (Y/N):

Type of deceleration:

Answers

Heart rate: Indeterminate

FHR category: II

Variability: Indeterminate

Acceleration (Y/N): N

Deceleration (Y/N): Y

Type of deceleration: Variable

Nursing interventions include the following:

- Reposition the patient.
- Administer an IV fluid bolus (normal saline or lactated Ringer's solution).
- Administer oxygen.
- Encourage pushing every second or third contraction to allow for fetal oxygenation.
- If the FHR remains the same, the provider should be notified.

Case Study 7.19

A 29-year-old patient at 40+1 weeks' gestation has been in labor for 28 hours and has not received any opioids. The FHR has been category II for more than 10 hours. The FHR tracing is shown in Figure 7.19. What nursing interventions, if any, are needed?

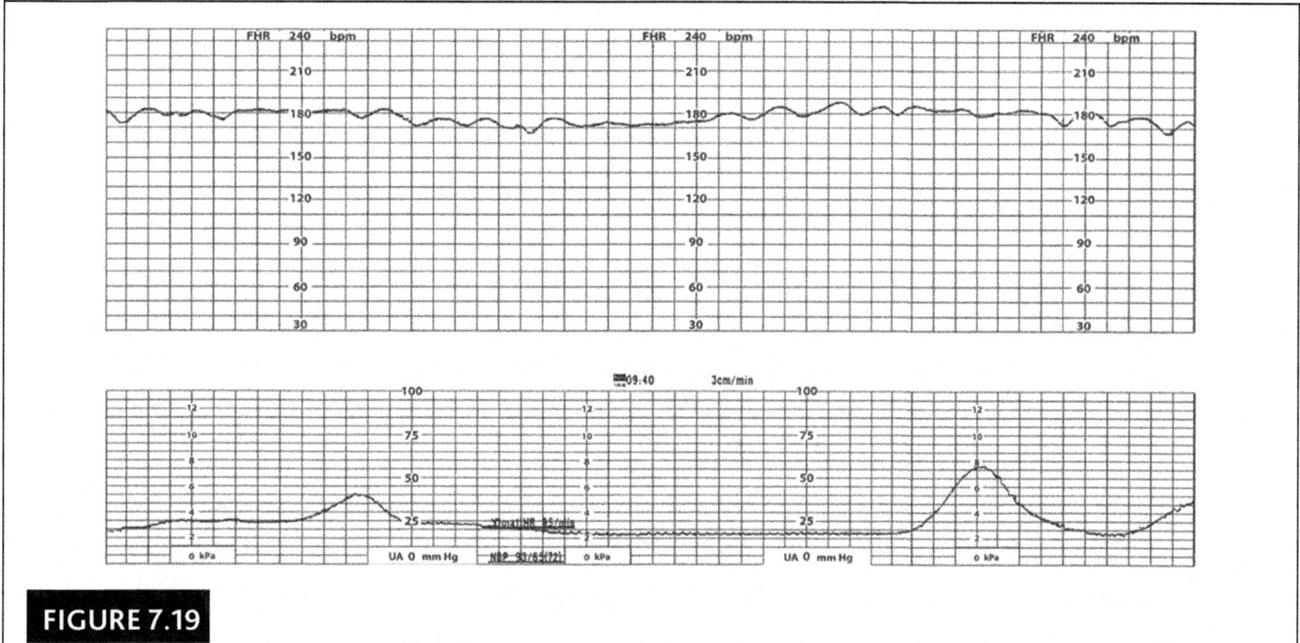

FIGURE 7.19

Source: Murray, M., Huelsmann, G., & Koperski, N. (2019). *Essentials of fetal and uterine monitoring* (5th ed.). Springer Publishing Company.

Heart rate:
FHR category:
Variability:
Acceleration (Y/N):
Deceleration (Y/N):
Type of deceleration:

Answers
Heart rate: 180
FHR category: II
Variability: N/A
Acceleration (Y/N): N
Deceleration (Y/N): N
Type of deceleration: None
The FHR reveals a sinusoidal pattern and requires immediate attention. The nurse should do the following:

- Call the provider.
- Start an IV.
- Administer an IV fluid bolus (normal saline or lactated Ringer's solution).
- Administer oxygen.

Case Study 7.20

The nurse performs all of the interventions described in Case Study 7.19. The tracing remains the same. What can the nurse expect to occur next?

Answer

The nurse can expect the provider to perform a cesarean section if vaginal delivery is not immediately pending.

RESOURCES

Garite, T. J., & Simpson, K. R. (2011). Intrauterine resuscitation during labor. *Clinical Obstetrics & Gynecology, 54*(1), 28–39. https://doi.org/10.1097/grf.0b013e31820a062b

Lakhno, I., Behar, J. A., Oster, J., Shulgin, V., Ostras, O., & Andreotti, F. (2017). The use of non-invasive fetal electrocardiography in diagnosing second-degree fetal atrioventricular block. *Maternal Health, Neonatology and Perinatology, 3*, Article 14. https://doi.org/10.1186/s40748-017-0053-1

Murray, M., Huelsmann, G., & Koperski, N. (2019). *Essentials of fetal and uterine monitoring* (5th ed.). Springer Publishing Company.

National Certification Corporation. (2021). *Fetal assessment and safe labor management*. https://www .nccwebsite.org/content/documents/cms/2016_ncc_monograph_free_version.pdf

Nye, R. (2019). *Essentials of fetal heart rate monitoring*. Springer Publishing Company.

PRACTICE TEST QUESTIONS

1. A patient is admitted in spontaneous labor 6 cm/100% effacement/0 station, with spontaneous rupture of the membranes and monitored with an internal uterine pressure catheter and fetal EKG. The nurse notes that over the past 20 minutes, the uterine contractions are 1 to 2 minutes apart, 80 to 100 seconds in duration, with a strength of 50 to 75 mmHg, and a resting tone of 15 to 20 mmHg. The fetal heart rate baseline is 145 bpm, minimal variability, with periodic variables and late decelerations present. After initiating intrauterine resuscitation measures, the nurse will plan to:
   A. Administer a tocolytic
   B. Prepare for fetal blood scalp sampling
   C. Prepare the patient for delivery

2. If the fetal Po_2 falls below a critical level, chemoreceptors trigger a sympathetic response, causing vasoconstriction of the peripheral blood vessels, prompting a rise in mean arterial pressure. This physiologic event results in a fetal heart rate:
   A. Decrease
   B. Increase
   C. Stabilization

3. A rise in fetal arterial pressure leads to:
   A. Decreased heart rate
   B. Increased heart rate
   C. Increased variability

4. The nurse observing a tracing of a laboring patient notes the fetal heart rate baseline is 140 bpm, moderate variability is present with decelerations that are symmetrical in shape, have a 40-second onset to the nadir, and last 60 seconds occurring simultaneously with contractions. There are no accelerations. The nurse will document the category of tracing as a:
   A. Category I
   B. Category II
   C. Category III

5. If all fetal heart rate (FHR) components are normal, the FHR tracing reliably predicts the absence of fetal metabolic acidemia and ongoing hypoxic injury and is documented as a:
   A. Category I FHR tracing
   B. Category II FHR tracing
   C. Category III FHR tracing

6. A woman G2P0 36 4/7 weeks is being induced for preeclampsia. The results of the amniocentesis performed earlier shows a lecithin-to-sphingomyelin ratio greater than 2.0. The respiratory distress syndrome risk assessment for this neonate is categorized as:
   A. High
   B. Minimal
   C. Moderate

7. The most accurate statement regarding a nonstress test (NST) on a patient at 39 weeks' gestation is a(n):
   A. Nonreactive NST is diagnostic of fetal hypoxia
   B. NST has a high predictive value for determining fetal hypoxia
   C. Reactive NST has a high negative predictive value of stillbirth within 1 week of testing

8. The nurse notes a fetal heart rate tracing has a baseline of 155 bpm, minimal variability, and variable decelerations that contain overshoots. This finding can be interpreted as:
   A. A fetal sleep cycle
   B. Fetal compensation
   C. Umbilical vein compression

9. Thirty minutes ago, the nurse administered butorphanol to a laboring patient 5 cm/80% effaced/−1 station, with intact membranes. Over the past 20 minutes, two fetal heart rate decelerations, 25 beats below the baseline for 2½ and 3 minutes occurred. The patient has contractions every 3 minutes, 40 to 70 seconds in duration, with adequate resting tone. After repositioning the patient, the nurse will:
   A. Administer a tocolytic
   B. Assess the maternal blood pressure
   C. Perform a vaginal examination

10. A factor that MOST influences the nurse's ability to provide safe patient care is:
    A. Attendance at mandatory unit meetings
    B. Interpersonal stress
    C. Number of continuing education contact hours obtained

11. The nurse reviewing a laboring patient's fetal heart rate (FHR) tracing notes a baseline of 115 bpm, with FHR fluctuations to 100 bpm for 25 seconds returning to the baseline 40 seconds after the contractions. Based on the interpretation of the tracing, the nurse will:
    A. Apply a fetal scalp electrode
    B. Assess the patient's cervical dilation
    C. Implement intrauterine resuscitation measures

12. The nurse notes that a fetus is experiencing bradycardia during the second stage of labor. The nurse understands the difference between recognizing hypoxic and nonhypoxic bradycardia is:
    A. Absence of periodic changes
    B. Presence of early decelerations
    C. Type of variability present

13. When the chart paper speed of the fetal monitor is set at 2 cm/min, the nurse can expect the FHR tracing to appear:
    A. Compressed
    B. Expanded
    C. Unaltered

14. The nurse is caring for a patient at 33 weeks' gestation admitted with influenza, with a heart rate of 88 bpm, temperature of 100.4°F (38.0°C), blood pressure of 148/76 mmHg, and respiratory rate of 20 per minute. The fetal heart rate baseline is 160 bpm, with minimal variability and absent accelerations. Immediately after initiating intrauterine resuscitation measures, the nurse will:
    A. Apply scalp stimulation
    B. Continue to monitor the fetus
    C. Prepare the patient for delivery

15. The nurse observing a fetal heart rate (FHR) tracing notes the FHR baseline is 108 bpm. A tracing denoting this baseline is:
    A. A fairly common occurrence
    B. Generally associated with minimal variability
    C. Not always associated with decreased oxygenation

16. Prior to conducting a nonstress test, the nurse will consider factors that affect fetal movement patterns, such as:
    A. Distended bladder
    B. Maternal hydration
    C. Twin gestation

17. The nurse is preparing to assess the fetal heart rate pattern of a patient who has received an opioid analgesic. The type of variability the nurse can expect to see is:
    A. Marked
    B. Minimal
    C. Moderate

18. While reviewing external monitoring tracing during labor, the nurse becomes concerned about fetal hypoxia. An intervention the nurse will implement to assess the fetus is:
    A. Fetal scalp sampling
    B. Scalp stimulation
    C. Vibroacoustic stimulation

19. The tocodynamometer is placed on the abdomen over the uterine:
    A. Cervix
    B. Fundus
    C. Lower segment

20. The nurse is caring for a patient who developed hypotension after receiving regional anesthesia. The episodic changes in the fetal heart rate pattern the nurse will closely monitor the patient for are:
    A. Late decelerations
    B. Prolonged accelerations
    C. Variables with overshoots

21. A medication associated with decreased reactivity and blunted responses to vibroacoustic stimulation is:
    A. Acetaminophen
    B. Magnesium sulfate
    C. Terbutaline

22. The nurse notes a fetal heart rate tracing has a baseline of 180 bpm. The potential cause of the baseline is:
    A. Administration of methyldopa
    B. Fetal heart block
    C. Maternal hyperthyroidism

23. When monitoring the uterine activity of a patient with minimal subcutaneous abdominal tissue with a tocotransducer, the nurse can anticipate:
    A. A blunt appearance of the uterine activity
    B. A prominent appearance of the uterine activity
    C. Difficulty obtaining a tracing of the uterine activity

24. The nurse evaluating the fetal heart rate (FHR) tracing of a patient at 37 weeks' gestation notes the FHR baseline to be 120 bpm during the first 10 minutes with absent variability and recurring late decelerations. The nurse will anticipate:
    A. Applying scalp stimulation
    B. Preparing the patient for a biophysical profile
    C. Preparing the patient for delivery

25. The nurse observes the fetal heart rate baseline over a 20-minute period to be between 128 and 136 bpm. To begin calculating the mean, the nurse will first:
    A. Add the two numbers
    B. Divide the two numbers
    C. Subtract the two numbers

26. The nurse is preparing to identify the category of variability of a fetal heart rate (FHR) tracing. The nurse understands that variability refers to:
    A. An interval that elapses between heartbeats
    B. Changes in the FHR baseline over a period of time
    C. Fluctuations in the FHR baseline

27. The accuracy of fetal assessment methods improve when electronic fetal heart rate monitoring is accompanied by:
   A. Amniocentesis
   B. Kick counts
   C. Ultrasound technology

28. The nurse notes a patient has a sinusoidal fetal heart rate pattern. The nurse understands that the component of the tracing that cannot be evaluated is:
   A. The baseline
   B. Decelerations
   C. The variability

29. Acute hypotension stimulates a response in the arterial baroreceptors resulting in:
   A. Fetal bradycardia
   B. Release of bicarbonate
   C. Vasoconstriction

30. The nurse will consider calculating the mean fetal heart rate (FHR) baseline when:
   A. The recorded FHR is sporadic
   B. The tracing exceeds 10 minutes
   C. There is less than 10 minutes of a tracing

31. The nurse understands that the interpretation of the fetal heart rate (FHR) baseline is subjective because:
   A. It is based on visual assessment
   B. The FHR baseline is constantly changing
   C. There are no guidelines for interpretation

32. An iatrogenic cause of decreased uterine blood flow is:
   A. Chronic hypertension
   B. Regional anesthesia
   C. Spontaneous tachysystole

33. A uterus that maintains a pressure of less than 20 mmHg remains below the level for concern of:
   A. Hypertonus
   B. Tachysystole
   C. Tetany

34. Scalp stimulation should be performed:
   A. As a component of intrauterine resuscitation
   B. During a deceleration
   C. When the fetal heart rate is at baseline and in between decelerations

35. The nurse is preparing to assess the fetal heart rate baseline during a 10-minute segment. To obtain the most accurate interpretation, the nurse will:
A. Determine the integers where the bulk of the data is contained
B. Note the highest and lowest points during the segment
C. Start at the beginning of the segment of tracing and note the changes throughout

36. Lateral positioning helps promote oxygenation by mechanically positioning the uterus off the:
A. Aorta or inferior vena cava
B. Diaphragm
C. Umbilical cord

37. The nurse has obtained a 20-minute tracing from a patient at 36 weeks' gestation reflecting the pattern shown. Based on this finding, the nurse will:

A. Continue to monitor the patient
B. Palpate the uterine activity
C. Place the patient in a lateral position

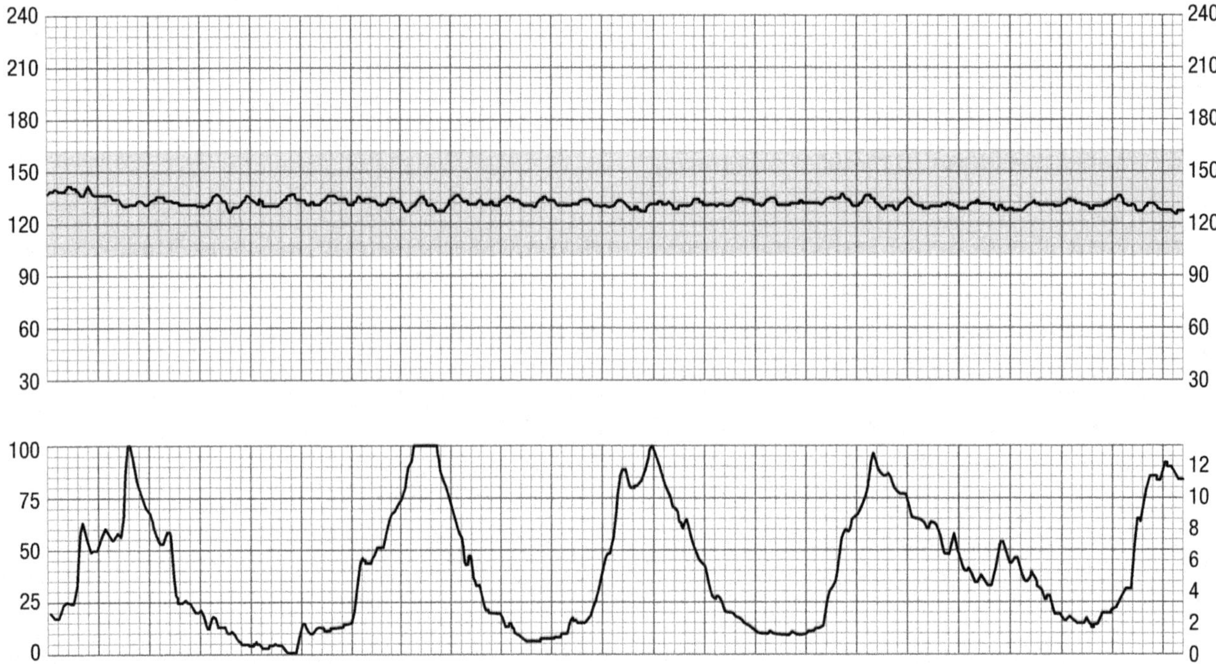

38. A woman at 35 weeks' gestation has a biophysical profile score of 6/10. The nurse will plan to:
A. Implement a contraction stress test
B. Prepare the patient for delivery
C. Repeat the testing in 24 hours

39. The primary concern about fetal well-being during tachysystole is the possible deficiency of maternal–fetal exchange of respiratory gases due to:
A. Blood in the intervillous spaces remaining in stasis for longer
B. Physiologic stress to the fetus
C. The dilation of spiral arteries

40. A primary function of the fetal sympathetic nervous system is to:
   A. Conserve body energy
   B. Eliminate body waste
   C. Prepare for stressful situations

41. The nurse is preparing to monitor a patient at 36 weeks' gestation who has a fetus with a neural tube defect. The nurse can anticipate the fetal heart rate variability on the tracing to be:
   A. Indeterminant
   B. Marked
   C. Minimal

42. A finding the nurse will anticipate in the fetal heart rate baseline of a well-oxygenated fetus is:
   A. Consistency of the heart rate
   B. Minimal changes in the heart rate
   C. Significant changes in the heart rate

43. Marked variability is defined as fluctuation of the fetal heart rate baseline of:
   A. Between 6 and 25 bpm
   B. Greater than 25 bpm
   C. Less than 6 bpm

44. The nurse monitoring a patient in the second stage of labor, who is pushing while lying on her left side, is obtaining a tracing using a fetal EKG and intrauterine pressure catheter. Based on the nurse's inability to interpret the fetal heart rate baseline or the type of decelerations present over the past 15 minutes, the nurse will:
   A. Change the position of the patient
   B. Encourage the patient to push with every other contraction
   C. Instruct the patient to stop pushing

45. The nurse observes intermittent early decelerations on a fetal heart rate tracing. The finding indicates that early decelerations occur with the uterine contractions over a 20-minute window less than:
   A. 30% of the time
   B. 40% of the time
   C. 50% of the time

46. The nurse calculates the mean fetal heart rate to be 153 bpm. The nurse should record the baseline rate as:
   A. 150
   B. 153
   C. 155

47. After applying oxygen to a patient with a category II tracing, the nurse asks the preceptor why a nonrebreather mask is used instead of a nasal cannula. The preceptor's best response is:

    A. "Maternal hyperoxia has not been associated with any negative outcomes or potential risks."

    B. "Nasal cannula administration of oxygen is associated with more cases of hyperoxia and damage due to free radicals."

    C. "The method that provides the highest fraction of inspired oxygen to the mother should be used when intervening on a nonreassuring fetal heart rate. The nonrebreather has the highest FIO_2 available for oxygen administration over the nasal cannula and simple face mask."

48. Fetal bradycardia is nonhypoxic when:

    A. Moderate variability is present

    B. Uterine activity is absent

    C. The baseline is above 100 bpm

49. The nurse observes a fetal heart rate tracing with a bradycardic baseline and minimal variability. The nurse will prepare to:

    A. Apply vibroacoustic stimulation

    B. Perform a vaginal examination

    C. Place the patient in a lateral position

50. Based on the interpretation of this tracing, the pattern would be documented as:

    A. Indeterminate

    B. Pseudo-sinusoidal

    C. Sinusoidal

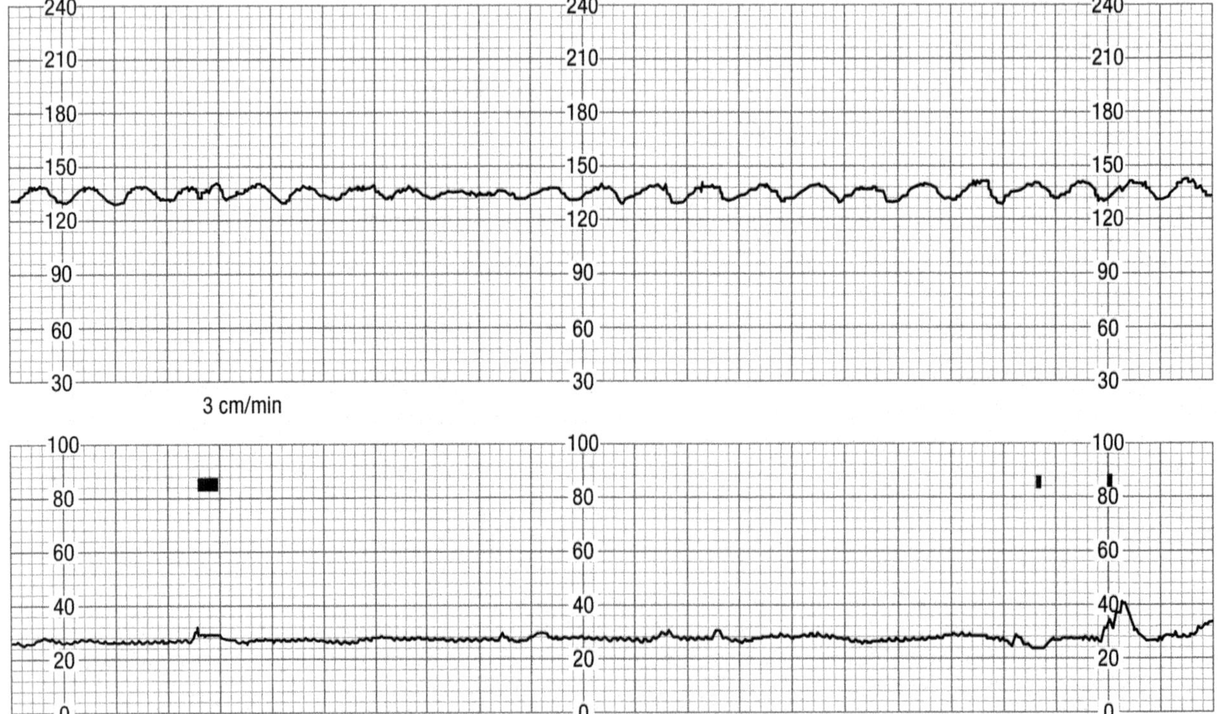

51. The nurse notes that a laboring patient has a fetal heart rate baseline of 105 bpm. To help determine the fetus is not hypoxic, the nurse will correlate the baseline with the:
   A. Gestational age
   B. Stage of labor
   C. Variability

52. The intrauterine pressure catheter provides an absolute measurement of intra-amniotic pressure because it:
   A. Has a fluid-filled sensor tip
   B. Houses a sensor that can detect myometrial tone
   C. Is referenced to atmospheric pressure

53. The nurse is preparing to determine the fetal heart rate (FHR) baseline of a fetus at 36 weeks' gestation. When evaluating the FHR baseline, the nurse will:
   A. Exclude FHR accelerations
   B. Evaluate the baseline over 20 minutes
   C. Round to increments of 10

54. The nurse receiving a report about a laboring patient is informed the fetal heart rate (FHR) baseline is bradycardic. The FHR baseline the nurse will associate with the report is:
   A. 105 bpm
   B. 115 bpm
   C. 125 bpm

55. The nurse is reviewing the maternal health history of the patients on the unit. The nurse recognizes that the patient most at risk for diminished placental function is:
   A. The patient who smokes
   B. The patient with cervical incompetence
   C. The patient with multiple gestations

56. A fetal heart rate (FHR) tracing denotes tachysystole. A type of FHR deceleration that this pattern can cause is:
   A. Early
   B. Prolonged
   C. Variable

57. The normal fetal metabolic process begins as:
   A. Carbon dioxide is removed
   B. Glucose is broken down
   C. Oxygen is delivered to the fetus

58. The nurse observing a nonstress test tracing notes a baseline of 135 bpm, moderate variability, two accelerations, and repetitive variable decelerations over a 20-minute time frame. The nurse will anticipate preparing the patient for a(n):
    A. Contraction stress test
    B. Ultrasound
    C. Vibroacoustic stimulation

59. When observing a fetal heart rate tracing on a central monitor display, the nurse understands that:
    A. The information is very accurate
    B. The strip chart at the bedside will look completely different
    C. There may be a discrepancy between the monitor and strip chart

60. The nurse notes a normal uterine pattern on the FHR tracing. The nurse understands that the maximum number of contractions that can occur within 10 minutes is:
    A. Four
    B. Five
    C. Six

61. On the tracing of a fetus at 37 weeks' gestation the nurse notes a baseline of 140 bpm, moderate variability, and abrupt fetal heart rate (FHR) decelerations 25 beats below the baseline lasting 30 seconds before returning to the baseline. The uterine activity recorded on the tracing is unclear. The nurse will document the FHR decelerations as:
    A. Episodic late
    B. Indeterminate variable
    C. Periodic early

62. The nurse notes a fetal heart rate tracing that has a normal baseline and marked variability. The nurse understands that when marked variability is present it:
    A. Is associated with fetal hypoxia
    B. Is a reassuring sign
    C. Requires further patient evaluation

63. The nurse is caring for a laboring patient 4 cm/75% effacement/–1 station, ruptured membranes with clear fluid, receiving oxytocin 10 milliunits/min. The fetal heart rate (FHR) tracing denotes a baseline of 140 bpm, minimal FHR variability, and intermittent late decelerations. The patient's contractions are 2 to 4 minutes apart, 40 to 60 seconds in duration, moderate to palpation, and adequate resting tone in between. Based on these findings, the nurse will:
    A. Continue to monitor the patient
    B. Discontinue the oxytocin
    C. Prepare the patient for delivery

64. The cell type of the placenta that is responsible for filtering nutrients and waste products between the maternal and fetal systems is the:
    A. Chorionic villi
    B. Fetal trophoblast
    C. Intervillous space

65. The nurse notes the presence of uniform accelerations on a fetal heart rate tracing. The nurse recognizes that this pattern usually occurs in response to:
    A. Mild cord compression
    B. Second stage of labor
    C. Uteroplacental insufficiency

66. The nurse observes a fetal heart rate pattern that has absent variability. An additional finding on the tracing necessary to classify it as a category III tracing is:
    A. Fetal tachycardia
    B. Pseudo-sinusoidal pattern
    C. Recurrent variable decelerations

67. The nurse notes the fetal heart rate (FHR) baseline of a fetus at 37 weeks' gestation has risen by 15 beats. The minimal duration of the increase in the FHR that must be present for it to be considered an acceleration is:
    A. 10 seconds
    B. 15 seconds
    C. 20 seconds

68. A factor related to the development of uterine tachysystole is:
    A. Epidural analgesia
    B. Fetal movement
    C. Maternal hypotension

69. The new nurse manager notes that there has been no validated competency for the nursing staff for the past 3 years. This is an example of a(n):
    A. Ethical dilemma
    B. Patient safety issue
    C. Quality improvement dilemma

70. The nurse is caring for a laboring patient contracting every 2 to 4 minutes with periodic variables and late decelerations. In relation to the contraction, the best time for the nurse to evaluate the fetal heart rate baseline is:
    A. During
    B. Immediately after
    C. Immediately before

71. A patient presents to the labor and delivery unit with symptoms of constant abdominal pain, and the uterus is rigid to palpation. Based on the assessment findings, the nurse suspects placental abruption and will anticipate the fetal heart rate tracing to denote:
    A. Early decelerations
    B. Prolonged accelerations
    C. Sinusoidal pattern

72. The nurse is reviewing the characteristics of fetal dysrhythmias. The nurse understands that most fetal dysrhythmias are recognizable on a strip chart as abrupt changes in the:
    A. Baseline
    B. Rhythm
    C. Variability

73. The primary intervention for variable decelerations is to:
    A. Continue to observe the patient
    B. Decrease any oxytocin infusions that may be occurring
    C. Reposition the patient

74. When monitoring an extremely preterm fetus, the nurse will consider:
    A. Affirming the presence of a fetal heart rate with a handheld Doppler
    B. Applying the external monitor to the middle of the abdomen
    C. Planning for continuous adjustment of the external monitor

75. Application of vibroacoustic stimulation is most effective when placed over:
    A. Either the fetal vertex or breech
    B. The fetal breech
    C. The fetal vertex

76. A component of a normal contraction pattern includes:
    A. Contraction strength of 80 to 100 mmHg
    B. The duration of the contractions to be 90 to 120 seconds
    C. Three to five contractions every 10 minutes

77. The nurse is monitoring a fetus at 27 weeks' gestation. The type of variability the nurse can anticipate is:
    A. Absent
    B. Marked
    C. Minimal

78. The nurse is evaluating the results of an umbilical arterial cord gas. The nurse understands that the balance of hydrogen (H^+) and hydroxyl (OH^-) ions:
    A. Affects fetal oxygenation
    B. Determines the pH
    C. Reflects the $PaCO_2$

79. When a fetus is unable to excrete nonvolatile acid in utero, the nurse can anticipate:

A. Decreased fetal movement

B. Increased fetal breathing

C. Increased fetal tone

80. After a fetal heart rate tracing is deemed nonreassuring, the decision is made to perform a Cesarean section to expedite delivery. Surgery should be initiated:

A. As soon as possible

B. Once the support person arrives

C. Within 30 minutes

81. While reviewing the fetal heart rate (FHR) tracing of a laboring patient, the nurse notes that the FHR over a 20-minute period ranges from 146 to 160 bpm and contains accelerations that rise 15 beats above the baseline for 20 seconds. The nurse will document the baseline as:

A. 150 bpm

B. 155 bpm

C. 160 bpm

82. The nurse is reviewing the first nonstress test of a patient with type 1 diabetes at 31 weeks' gestation, scheduled for weekly testing. After 20 minutes of monitoring, the tracing denotes a fetal heart rate baseline of 140 bpm, minimal variability, and two accelerations 5 beats above the baseline for 10 seconds. Based on the interpretation of the tracing, the nurse will:

A. Ask the patient if they have taken their daily insulin

B. Ask the patient if they recently had anything to eat or drink

C. Instruct the patient to return to the clinic in a week

83. The nurse notes periodic variable decelerations on the fetal heart rate (FHR) tracing of a patient in labor. To help resolve the FHR pattern, the nurse will:

A. Administer oxygen to the patient

B. Perform scalp stimulation

C. Reposition the patient

84. A healthcare provider tells the nurse who is caring for a patient with a nonreassuring tracing to discharge the patient home. The nurse will:

A. Activate the chain of command

B. Contact the ethics committee

C. Discharge the patient home

85. During the bolus and maintenance of an amnioinfusion, the returning amount of fluid should be noted and recorded to avoid causing iatrogenic:

A. Oligohydramnios

B. Polyhydramnios

C. Tachysystole

86. The nurse is reviewing a list of patients in the labor and delivery unit. The laboring patient likely to have a tracing with late decelerations is:
    A. A patient at 34 weeks' gestation in premature labor
    B. A patient in active labor who has received nalbuphine
    C. A patient with type 1 diabetes in spontaneous labor

87. The final step the nurse will take when interpreting the fetal heart rate (FHR) pattern is to assess the FHR:
    A. Baseline
    B. Responses
    C. Variability

88. The nurse is evaluating a fetal heart rate baseline. The nurse will exclude:
    A. Marked variability
    B. Minimal variability
    C. Moderate variability

89. The nurse is caring for a laboring patient G1 P0, who 1 hour prior was 9 cm/100% effaced, +1 station, and ruptured membranes with clear fluid. The patient's contractions are every 2 to 3 minutes, 60 to 70 seconds in duration, moderate to palpation, with adequate resting tone. The fetal heart rate baseline is 145 bpm, showing moderate variability with the presence of intermittent late decelerations. The nurse will:
    A. Assess cervical dilation
    B. Continue to monitor the patient
    C. Place the patient in a lateral position

90. A benefit of using a written examination to validate staff competency is that:
    A. An examination can be used for multiple disciplines
    B. Any team member can devise an exam
    C. It is a recognized tool to validate competency

91. Based on the interpretation of this tracing, the variability would be documented as:
   A. Absent
   B. Marked
   C. Moderate

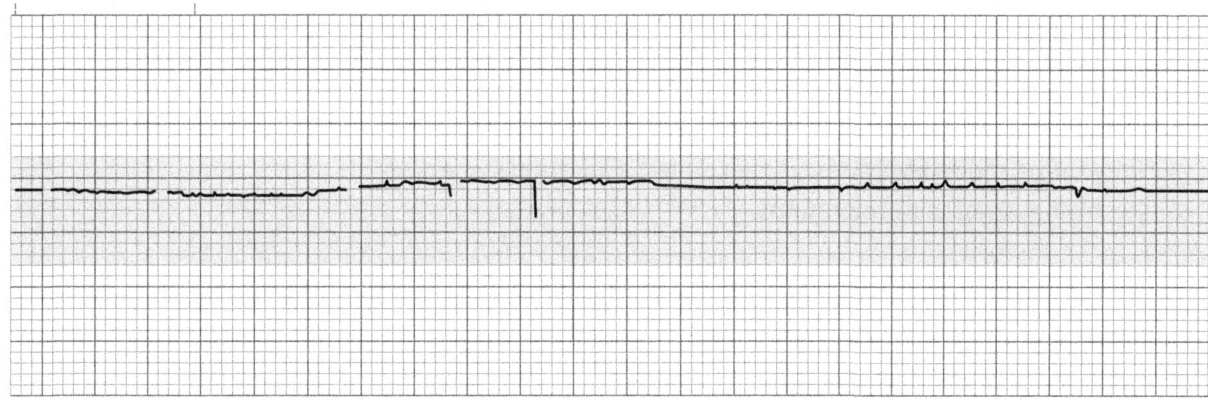

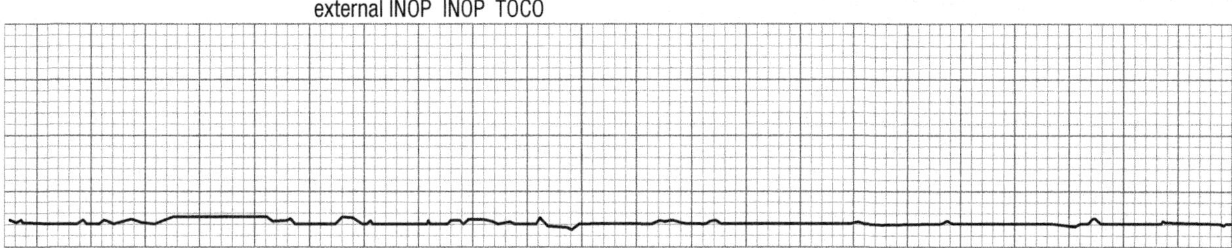

92. A woman at 34 weeks' gestation who had a modified biophysical profile (BPP) has a reactive nonstress test and an amniotic fluid index greater than 4 cm. The nurse will presume another component of a BPP that is adequate is:
   A. Fetal breathing
   B. Fetal growth
   C. Fetal tone

93. The nurse is preparing to monitor a fetus at 31 weeks' gestation. The fetal heart rate beats above the baseline associated with accelerations that the nurse can anticipate are:
   A. 5
   B. 10
   C. 15

94. The nurse is monitoring a patient at 27 weeks' gestation for decreased fetal movement. The tracing reveals a 20-minute pattern of baseline variability and no accelerations. The nurse will plan to:
   A. Continue to monitor the patient
   B. Discontinue monitoring the patient
   C. Prepare the patient for a biophysical profile

95. The nurse has applied an internal fetal monitor to a fetus with a dysrhythmia. The type of variability the nurse can anticipate is:
    A. Marked
    B. Minimal
    C. Moderate

96. Amnioinfusion has been shown to be effective in:
    A. Delaying active labor
    B. Preventing moderate to severe meconium aspiration syndrome
    C. Resolving variable decelerations

97. To shorten the testing time and reduce the number of nonreassuring results of a biophysical profile, the nurse will:
    A. Implement acoustic stimulation
    B. Omit the nonstress test
    C. Perform a contraction stress test

98. The nurse reviewing a fetal heart rate tracing observes repetitive late decelerations. The nurse should associate this pattern with:
    A. Fetal hypoxia
    B. Fetal sleep
    C. Umbilical cord compression

99. During labor, the fetal heart rate is interpreted in conjunction with:
    A. A biophysical profile
    B. Fetal movement
    C. Uterine activity

100. The first change noted in the components of a biophysical profile scoring for a fetus initially experiencing hypoxia is:
    A. Absent fetal movement
    B. Decreased fetal breathing movements
    C. Loss of fetal heart rate activity

101. The nurse monitoring a fetus with a fetal scalp electrode (FSE) cannot tell the difference between artifact and dysrhythmia in the fetal heart rate (FHR) pattern. The nurse will:
    A. Auscultate the FHR with a handheld Doppler
    B. Perform a vaginal examination to determine the placement of the FSE
    C. Replace the FSE with an external monitor

102. Based on the interpretation of this tracing, the variability would be documented as:
- A. Marked
- B. Minimal
- C. Moderate

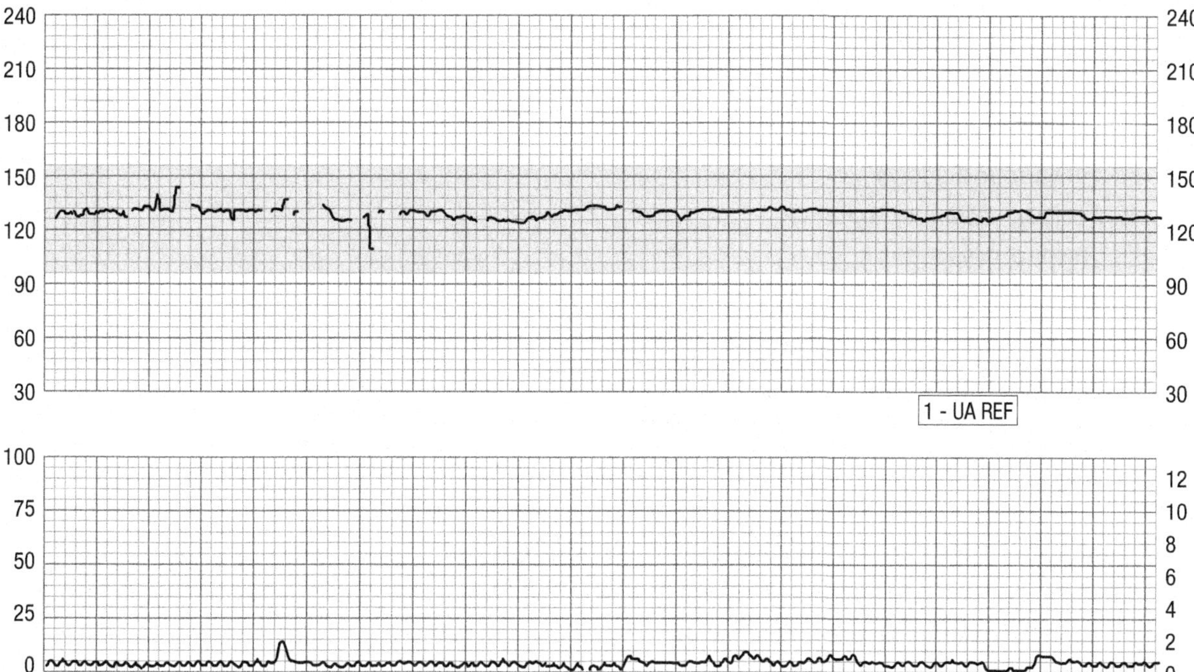

103. A risk of blood type incompatibility between mother and fetus during an amniocentesis is:
- A. Alloimmunization
- B. Bleeding
- C. Infection

104. Early decelerations are associated with:
- A. A disruption of oxygenation
- B. Maternal administration of narcotic analgesics
- C. Transient fetal head compression

105. Uterine activity is determined by the number of contractions present in a 10-minute window:
- A. Averaged after 10 minutes
- B. Averaged after 30 minutes
- C. Multiplied by 2

106. The nurse educator discusses the scope of practice with a new nurse in the labor and delivery unit. When discussing the nurse's response to fetal heart rate changes, the nurse educator will note:
- A. "All nursing interventions are dependent."
- B. "Nurses implement independent interventions."
- C. "The ability to implement interventions is based on state Nurse Practice Act."

107. Scalp stimulation should be avoided in:
   A. A G1P0 patient who has had a nonreactive nonstress test for over 20 minutes
   B. A G1P2 patient in active labor with fetus A
   C. A G3P1 patient who is 5/80/−2

108. The nurse reviewing the umbilical cord arterial gas from a fetus with a category II tracing notes the pH is 7.20, Po_2 is 20.8 mmHg, $Paco_2$ is 45.5 mmHg, and base excess is 9 mEq/L. The interpretation the nurse will report to the healthcare provider is:
   A. Metabolic acidosis
   B. Normal acid–base balance
   C. Respiratory acidosis

109. The nurse notes a fetal heart rate baseline is 175 bpm. A possible cause of this baseline is:
   A. Chorioamnionitis
   B. Electrical impulse reentering the ventricle
   C. Fetal hypothermia

110. Fetal pulse oximetry was concluded to be of limited usefulness after several randomized controlled trials in the presence of indeterminate or abnormal fetal heart tracings due to the technology:
   A. Being expensive despite its accuracy
   B. Failing to distinguish between maternal and fetal oxygenation
   C. Not reducing the overall Cesarean section rate and being exceedingly difficult to place

111. The nurse is reviewing the physiology of the blood flow through the uterine vessels. The uterine vascular bed:
   A. Changes based on the level of fetal oxygenation
   B. Is controlled by the central nervous system
   C. Constantly maintains maximum dilation

112. The nurse monitoring a patient in labor is concerned that the recording on the tracing is the maternal heart rate. The initial action the nurse should take is:
   A. Palpate the maternal pulse and compare it to the audible signal
   B. Perform Leopold's maneuver and reapply the external monitor
   C. Remove the external monitor and apply a fetal scalp electrode

113. The nurse is reviewing the tracing of a term fetus. The nurse will document the finding as:
    A. Fetal bradycardia
    B. Moderate variability
    C. Tracing is indeterminate

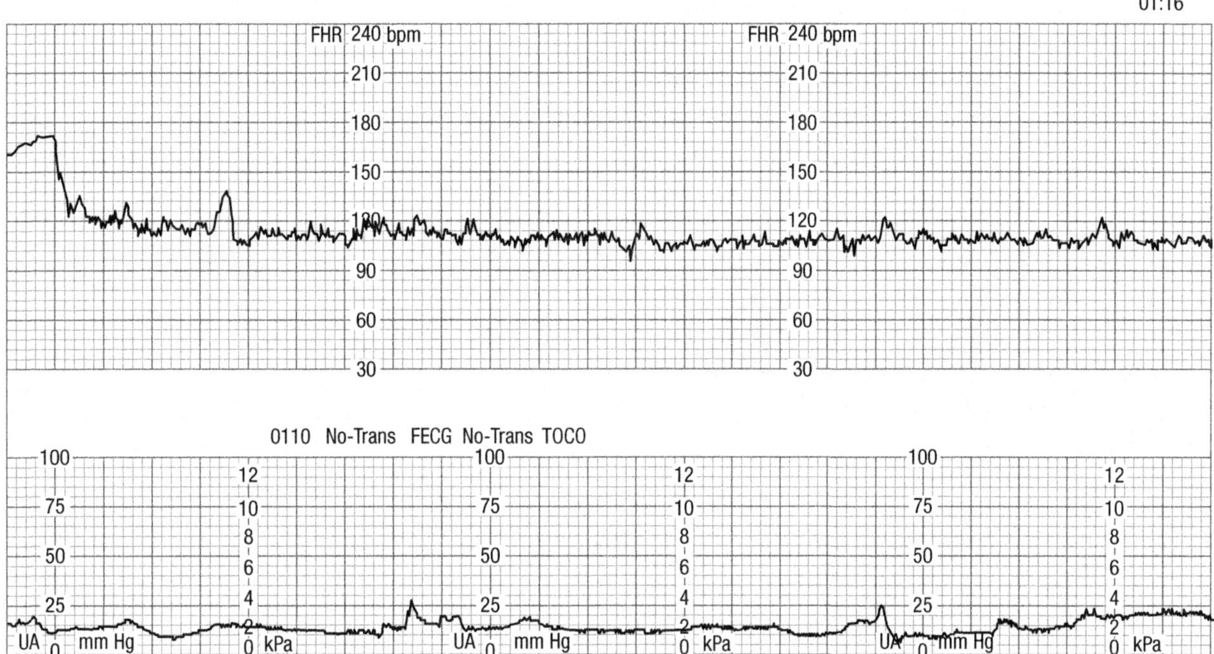

114. The nurse is reviewing the tracing of a term fetus with a pattern of supraventricular tachycardia. The most appropriate intervention for this condition is:
    A. Antiarrhythmic
    B. Atropine
    C. Beta-blocker

115. The nurse can safely perform a contraction stress test on a woman who is:
    A. 34 weeks' gestation with ruptured membranes not contracting
    B. 37 weeks' gestation with decreased fetal movement
    C. 38 weeks' gestation with a previous Cesarean section

116. The nurse manager has developed a medical record audit using guidelines and standards of care for a quality improvement project for the labor and delivery unit. The most accurate statement regarding the benefit of this audit is that it:
    A. Ensures that all skills are covered during orientation
    B. Is beneficial for new staff
    C. Promotes evidence-based practice

117. The nurse notes the fetal heart rate (FHR) tracing baseline is 165 bpm. In reference to the normal parameters of an FHR, the nurse understands that this finding is:
    A. Above
    B. Below
    C. Within

118. The nurse educator is preparing to validate the competence of a new nurse before completion of orientation. The nurse educator will:
    A. Administer a fetal heart rate pattern interpretation exam
    B. Audit the nurse's medical records
    C. Review the orientation checklist with the nurse

119. The nurse who is monitoring a fetus with a normal cardiac structure notes isolated extrasystoles on the tracing. The nurse recognizes that this finding is likely the result of:
    A. Abnormal fetal presentation
    B. Fetal sleep cycle
    C. Maternal intake of caffeine

120. When villi break off within the intervillous space, the nurse can expect:
    A. Exchange of maternal–fetal blood cells
    B. Fetal hyperglycemia
    C. Maternal immunoglobulins to enter the fetal system

121. The nurse is preparing to calculate the Montevideo units of a laboring patient. A component the nurse will include in the calculation is:
    A. Duration of the contractions
    B. Frequency of the contractions
    C. The strength of the contractions

122. The nurse caring for a laboring patient who is receiving oxytocin notes that over the last 30 minutes, the number of uterine contractions in a 10-minute period was seven. The nurse will:
    A. Increase the intravenous fluid
    B. Reposition the patient laterally
    C. Turn off the oxytocin

123. When aerobic metabolism is no longer effective, the fetal:
    A. Buffer system is activated
    B. Demand for oxygenation decreases
    C. pH increases

124. The most accurate statement regarding the contraction stress test (CST) is:
    A. The CST carries a high false-negative rate
    B. The CST is an earlier predictor of a deteriorating fetal status than a nonstress test
    C. The risk of fetal death within 72 hours is minimal when the CST is reassuring

125. The nurse notes a laboring patient has the following fetal heart rate pattern. The nurse recognizes this pattern as:

A. Indeterminant

B. Pseudo-sinusoidal

C. Sinusoidal

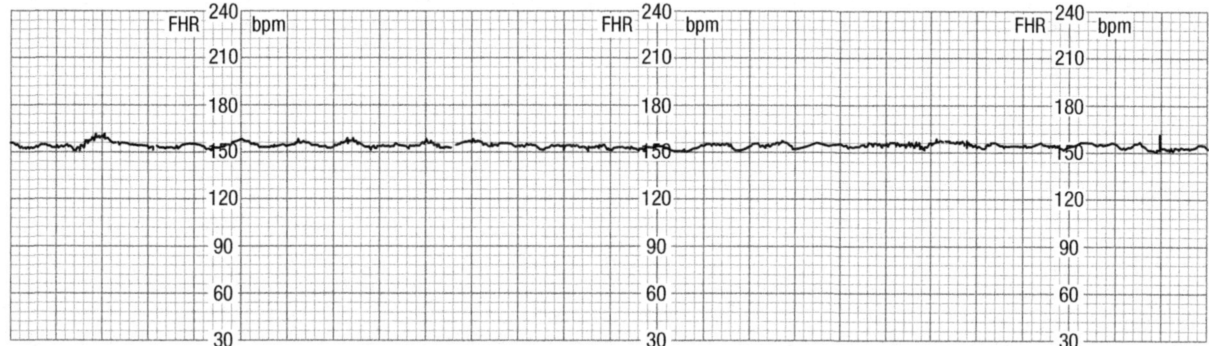

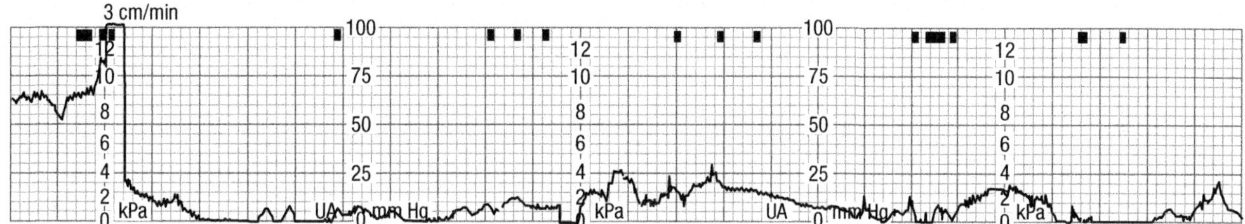

1. **A) Administer a tocolytic**
   For a patient with a category II tracing with uterine tachysystole whose fetus does not respond to intrauterine resuscitation measures, the nurse will plan to administer a tocolytic. The purpose of the tocolytic is to stop the tachysystole and allow the fetus to recover. Delivery is warranted if the fetal tracing becomes a category III. Fetal blood scalp sampling is invasive and is not frequently performed due to several limitations.

2. **A) Decrease**
   When peripheral vasoconstriction occurs, the fetal blood pressure rises dramatically. Baroreceptors monitoring for these changes respond immediately to increases in blood pressure by stimulating the parasympathetic system. The stimulation of the parasympathetic system slows the fetal heart rate to reduce cardiac output and return the blood pressure to normal. An increase in heart rate and peripheral vasoconstriction would increase blood pressure, which would continue to exacerbate fetal hypoxia. A significant drop below the vital oxygenation level causes the chemoreceptors to respond by altering the heart rate and blood pressure to achieve homeostasis.

3. **A) Decreased heart rate**
   When the arterial pressure rises in the fetus, the heart rate decreases, and vasodilation occurs to lower the arterial pressure. The fetal heart rate does not increase when the arterial pressure increases. Changes in variability are associated with compensatory mechanisms related to fetal oxygenation, such as tachycardia, in which the variability can be decreased.

4. **A) Category I**
   The fetal heart rate (FHR) is a category I tracing and is considered normal. The baseline is within the normal range of 110 to 160 bpm, and it has moderate variability, early decelerations, and absence of accelerations. Early decelerations result from compression of the fetal head during a contraction that stimulates the parasympathetic system. Early decelerations are not pathologic. A category II tracing will contain variable, late, or prolonged decelerations with minimal or moderate variability and is considered suspicious. An FHR tracing that is a category III has absent variability and recurrent variable or late decelerations, bradycardia, or a sinusoidal pattern.

5. **A) Category I FHR tracing**
   Category I refers to a normal fetal heart rate (FHR) tracing. Category II refers to an indeterminate FHR tracing. Category III refers to an abnormal FHR tracing.

6. B) Minimal

A lecithin-to-sphingomyelin (L/S) ratio greater than 2.0 indicates a low risk of neonatal surfactant deficient respiratory distress syndrome (RDS). Both moderate and high risks of RDS are associated with an L/S ratio of less than 2.0.

7. C) Reactive NST has a high negative predictive value of stillbirth within 1 week of testing

The nonstress test (NST) is used to evaluate the number of fetal heart rate accelerations within a 20-minute time frame. A reactive NST has a high negative predictive value of stillbirth within 1 week of testing. The NST is a screening tool, not a diagnostic tool, for evaluating fetal well-being; however, it has a poor predictive value for determining fetal hypoxia.

8. B) Fetal compensation

The compromised fetus, in an attempt to recover to the baseline rate, raises its heart rate well above the baseline after a variable deceleration. This process is called overshoot. When overshoots are present, variability in the fetal heart rate (FHR) baseline is usually minimal to absent, and there is no accelerative phase preceding the variable deceleration. The actual variable deceleration occurs as a result of umbilical cord compression. Shoulders are caused by umbilical vein compression. Shoulders are brief accelerations of the FHR that may immediately precede or follow the decelerative phase of the variable deceleration. Overshoots are not a finding associated with the fetal sleep cycle.

9. B) Assess the maternal blood pressure

The nurse will assess the maternal blood pressure. Butorphanol is an opioid agonist/antagonist that can cause hypotension. Maternal hypotension can interrupt maternal–fetal perfusion resulting in prolonged decelerations. Uterine tachysystole can cause prolonged decelerations, for which a tocolytic may be administered. However, the patient does not have uterine tachysystole. There is no indication a vaginal examination needs to be performed. A vaginal exam would be performed to rule out a cord prolapse if the patient's membranes were ruptured.

10. B) Interpersonal stress

Interpersonal stress can influence a nurse's ability to provide safe patient care. Other factors that can compromise patient safety include fatigue, staffing ratios, communication, and interaction with other providers. Continuing education and attendance at mandatory unit meetings can impact performance, but they are not factors that most influence a nurse's ability to provide safe patient care. Continuing education will help the nurse stay current with their knowledge to provide safe patient care, and mandatory staff meetings keep a nurse current on what changes are occurring on the unit.

11. C) Implement intrauterine resuscitation measures

The patient has late decelerations, which are a fetal reflex response to hypoxemia resulting from inadequate fetal oxygenation. The nurse will implement intrauterine resuscitation measures. Applying a fetal scalp electrode or assessing the patient's cervical dilation is unnecessary. The nurse's priority is to promote maternal–fetal perfusion.

12. C) Type of variability present

Bradycardia during the second stage of labor may be seen in an adequately oxygenated fetus as a normal response to vagal nerve stimulation. The key factor in recognizing the difference between hypoxic and nonhypoxic bradycardia during the second stage of labor is the fetal heart rate baseline variability. Bradycardia with absent or minimal variability is associated with hypoxia, whereas the variability will remain moderate in nonhypoxic instances. The absence of periodic changes or the presence of early decelerations are not key factors in recognizing the difference between hypoxic and nonhypoxic bradycardia.

13. A) Compressed

The general rate of paper speed in the United States is 3 cm/min. When the paper speed is set at 2 cm/min, the slower rate will cause the information on the tracing to appear compressed. The appearance of a tracing will be altered as the chart paper speed is adjusted. If the paper speed is set higher, the information will appear to be expanded.

14. B) Continue to monitor the fetus

The nurse will monitor the fetal response to the intrauterine resuscitation interventions. Maternal fever may result in dehydration, which can cause fetal tachycardia and decreased variability. There is no indication the fetus needs to be delivered. Delivery is indicated if the fetal condition deteriorates. Fetal scalp stimulation is not an appropriate action if fetal hypoxia is suspected.

15. C) Not always associated with decreased oxygenation

A baseline fetal heart rate that is inherently less than 110 bpm is rare and not always associated with decreased oxygenation. Fetal bradycardia can present with absent, minimal, and moderate variability. Fetal baseline bradycardia is uncommon.

16. B) Maternal hydration

Maternal hydration is a factor that affects fetal movement patterns. The fetus of a dehydrated woman will have decreased movement. Twin gestation and distended bladder do not affect fetal movement patterns.

17. B) Minimal

Medications that depress the maternal central nervous system (CNS) are expected to decrease the fetal heart rate variability because they have similar effects on the fetal CNS. Moderate variability can be expected to return when the medication is metabolized and excreted. Marked variability is not associated with the administration of an opioid analgesic. Marked variability can be associated with fetal activity or hypoxia.

18. B) Scalp stimulation

The external fetal monitor is not a good measure of fetal deoxygenation. The primary purpose of external fetal monitoring is to screen for hypoxia. Direct measures can be utilized in conjunction with external fetal monitoring to determine hypoxic fetuses from those with fetal heart rate tracings that are suspicious for hypoxia. Two adjuncts to external fetal monitoring include fetal scalp stimulation and vibroacoustic stimulation. Vibroacoustic stimulation is not performed during labor; therefore, the most appropriate intervention is scalp stimulation. Fetal scalp sampling is not frequently performed. The procedure is invasive, and it requires special training and laboratory testing, which a lab may not be able to perform.

19. B) Fundus

The fundus is the top and origin point for contractions of the uterus. It is the correct location for the tocodynamometer. The lower uterine segment is not associated with palpable contractions. The cervix is located internally and is not a location to monitor contractions.

20. A) Late decelerations

Maternal hypotension results in decreased blood flow to the placenta. Late decelerations can occur as a result of the decreased oxygenated blood flow to the fetus. Variable decelerations are caused by cord compression, not maternal hypotension. Prolonged accelerations are a sign of fetal well-being and the term is used to describe fetal heart rate accelerations with an amplitude of at least 15 bpm above the baseline lasting for at least 2 minutes but less than 10 minutes.

21. B) Magnesium sulfate

Magnesium sulfate is associated with blunted responses to vibroacoustic stimulation (VAS). A beta-agonist such as terbutaline or an analgesic such as acetaminophen is not associated with decreased reactivity or blunted VAS responses.

22. C) Maternal hyperthyroidism

Maternal hyperthyroidism is associated with fetal tachycardia. In rare cases, transplacental passage of thyroid-stimulating antibodies can result in fetal hyperthyroidism and tachycardia. Methyldopa is a sympatholytic used to treat hypertension. It can cause a decrease in the fetal heart rate. Fetal heart block is associated with bradycardia.

23. B) A prominent appearance of the uterine activity

The thickness of the patient's subcutaneous tissue can affect the tracing of the uterine activity. A patient with minimal subcutaneous tissue will have a prominent appearance of the uterine activity. A greater amount of subcutaneous tissue buffers the contraction from the tocotransducer, resulting in a blunt appearance of uterine activity. The nurse should not have difficulty obtaining a tracing of uterine activity for a patient with minimal subcutaneous tissue.

24. C) Preparing the patient for delivery

The combination of absent variability and recurring late decelerations reflects a category III tracing for which delivery is indicated. Undetectable fetal heart rate variability reflects a diminished blood flow to the placenta. Inadequate blood flow to the placenta results in decreased oxygenation to the fetus causing tissue hypoxia and metabolic acidosis. Late decelerations are a fetal reflex response to hypoxemia caused by insufficient maternal–fetal oxygenation. Applying scalp stimulation or preparing the patient for a biophysical profile are not appropriate actions; the priority is preparing the patient for delivery.

25. A) Add the two numbers

When calculating a mean baseline, the nurse will first add the two numbers together (128 + 136). The result of adding the numbers is then divided by 2 (264 ÷ 2 = 132). This number is rounded up to the nearest increment of 5 to obtain the baseline (132 becomes 135).

26. C) Fluctuations in the FHR baseline

Variability refers to fluctuations or changes in the fetal heart rate (FHR) baseline. An interval that elapses between heartbeats is a component of variability. Changes in the FHR baseline over a period refer to the consistency of the FHR baseline.

27. C) Ultrasound technology

Although electronic fetal heart rate (FHR) monitoring is a very sensitive tool for detecting interrupted fetal oxygenation via FHR patterns such as decelerations and decreased variability, the converse is not true; an oxygenated fetus can also display the same concerning FHR patterns. Ultrasound technology allows for the noninvasive assessment of fetal and placental status. The combination of electronic FHR monitoring with ultrasound technology allows for a more accurate assessment of both oxygenated and deoxygenated fetuses. Amniocenteses are performed to evaluate genetic abnormalities and lung maturity, not as markers for fetal well-being in conjunction with a nonstress test (NST). Kick counts are a subjective measurement of information that is objectively collected during an NST.

28. A) The baseline

When a sinusoidal pattern is present, the actual fetal heart rate (FHR) baseline is indeterminant. The variability of a sinusoidal pattern can be determined. The FHR variability is absent or minimal, giving the pattern its smooth shape. Decelerations such as late, variable, and prolonged can be present.

29. C) Vasoconstriction

Arterial baroreceptors are sensitive to the stretch or distention of a vessel that occurs with changes in blood pressure. Rapid decreases in blood pressure decrease stretching of the artery wall and action potential frequency. This causes an increase in cardiac output and vasoconstriction to increase blood pressure. A decrease in arterial pressure causes an increase in heart rate. The opposite is true for instances of increased blood pressure, which produces vessel distention. This causes arterial barorecep-tors to send neuronal messages to the cardioinhibitory center to decrease the fetal heart rate via the parasympathetic vagus nerve.

30. B) The tracing exceeds 10 minutes

The nurse needs a minimum of 10 minutes of tracing to interpret the baseline, but when the nurse eval-uates a larger time frame, a mean fetal heart rate (FHR) can be calculated. If the FHR is plotted over a visually wider range of time, it may be helpful to interpret the baseline by calculating the mean and then rounding it off. A sporadically recorded FHR tracing is not used to calculate an FHR baseline.

31. A) It is based on visual assessment

Interpretation of the fetal heart rate (FHR) baseline is subjective because it is based on visual assess-ment from individuals with varying degrees of experience and education. The interpretation of the FHR baseline is obtained by assessing 10 minutes of the tracing. This assessment is performed periodically to monitor for changes. Guidelines for interpretation and definitions are set forth by the National Institute of Child Health and Human Development (NICHD).

32. B) Regional anesthesia

Decreased uterine blood flow that is of an iatrogenic nature commonly occurs secondary to treatments and interventions. Regional anesthesia is an iatrogenic cause of decreased uterine blood flow. Chronic hypertension and spontaneous tachysystole are not considered iatrogenic causes of decreased uterine blood flow.

33. A) Hypertonus

Uterine tone is measured in mmHg and indicates the amount of muscle contraction that remains during the resting state. Tachysystole refers to greater than five contractions in a 10-minute period. Tetany describes a muscle during a prolonged contraction.

34. C) When the fetal heart rate is at baseline and in between decelerations

Scalp stimulation is performed to evaluate acid–base status in the setting of a category II or indeterminate fetal heart rate. Used during periods of decreased variability or the absence of spontaneous accelerations, these induced accelerations are associated with a pH of 7.19 or greater and the absence of acidosis. Scalp stimulation is not performed during decelerations. Scalp stimulation is not a component of intrauterine resuscitation. It is a method of assessing fetal acid–base status, not an intervention.

35. A) Determine the integers where the bulk of the data is contained

To critically evaluate the trend of the fetal heart rate data, the nurse will determine the integers between which the bulk of the data is contained. Once it is initially identified for that portion of the tracing, the nurse will reconfirm the finding at other points within the segment of tracing to ensure accuracy. Starting at the beginning of the tracing is not as effective as initially focusing on the bulk of the data.

36. A) Aorta or inferior vena cava

The aorta and inferior vena cava are at high risk of compression by the gravid uterus with supine positioning. Lateral positioning is performed to maximize maternal cardiac return and output to optimize blood flow to the uterus and placenta. The uterus location does not alter the function of the diaphragm. The umbilical cord is located within the uterus; therefore, it is impossible for the uterus to compress it.

37. B) Palpate the uterine activity

The tracing is suspicious for uterine tachysystole, which can cause prolonged decelerations, and requires close uterine monitoring, which can be done using palpation. Continuing to monitor the patient places the fetus at risk for hypoxia if uterine tachysystole is present and the fetus has prolonged decelerations. Placing the patient in a lateral position is necessary if the assessment findings indicate uterine tachysystole and prolonged fetal heart rate decelerations are present.

38. C) Repeat the testing in 24 hours

A biophysical profile (BPP) score of 6/10 is equivocal. A patient with an equivocal score should have the BPP repeated within 24 hours. A contraction stress test is not performed on a preterm patient. A BPP score of 6/10 does not indicate preparing the patient for delivery.

39. A) Blood in the intervillous spaces remaining in stasis for longer

Blood that is in the placenta and undergoing gas exchange is suspended from movement at the acme of uterine contractions. This moment is typically well tolerated by most fetuses unless risk factors like tachysystole are occurring. Frequent contractions can extend the time of stasis of blood flow which in turn inhibits gas exchange and fetal oxygenation. Physiologic stress to the fetus does not create deficiencies of the maternal–fetal exchange of respiratory gases. The spiral arteries do not dilate secondary to tachysystole.

40. C) Prepare for stressful situations

A primary function of the sympathetic nervous system is to prepare the body for stressful situations. Primary functions of the fetal parasympathetic nervous system include elimination of body waste and conservation of energy.

41. C) Minimal

A neural tube defect is an anomaly of the central nervous system (CNS) for which the nurse can anticipate minimal or absent variability. CNS anomalies affect the variability of the fetal heart rate. Marked variability is not a clinical finding associated with CNS anomalies. The variability can be determined for a fetus with a CNS anomaly.

42. A) Consistency of the heart rate

The nurse should anticipate a consistency in the fetal heart rate (FHR) baseline of a well-oxygenated fetus. Minimal rate changes in the heart rate refer to variability; however, this is not specifically an anticipated finding of a well-oxygenated fetus. Significant FHR baseline changes are not an anticipated finding for a well-oxygenated fetus.

43. B) Greater than 25 bpm

Marked variability is defined as a fluctuation in the fetal heart rate baseline of greater than 25 bpm. A fluctuation of less than 6 bpm is referred to as minimal variability. A fluctuation between 6 and 25 bpm is referred to as moderate variability.

44. C) Instruct the patient to stop pushing

The nurse will instruct the patient to stop pushing to improve fetal oxygenation until the pattern can be determined. Changing a patient's position from a lateral position may not be helpful because this position allows for improved maternal–fetal perfusion. Instructing the patient to push with every other contraction places the fetus at risk for further compromise. The nurse's priority is to accurately interpret the fetal heart rate tracing and ensure the fetus is adequately oxygenated.

45. C) 50% of the time

Intermittent early decelerations occur with contractions less than 50% of the time over a 20-minute window. The criteria for intermittent early decelerations are not less than 30% or 40% of the time.

46. C) 155

Once the mean heart rate is calculated, the nurse will round up that number to the nearest increment of 5. Therefore, a mean fetal heart rate (FHR) baseline of 153 bpm should be rounded to 155 bpm. An FHR baseline of 150 or 153 does not reflect an accurate interpretation of the baseline.

47. C) "The method that provides the highest fraction of inspired oxygen to the mother should be used when intervening on a nonreassuring FHR. The non rebreather has the highest FIO_2 available for oxygen administration over the nasal cannula and simple face mask."

The nonrebreather is the best option because the FIO_2 at 10 L/min is 80%–100%, which is much higher than with a simple face mask (27%–40%) or nasal cannula (31%). Free radicals are associated with higher levels of FIO_2. Maternal hyperoxia and hypoxia are associated with the production of oxygen free radicals capable of causing oxidative stress and damage.

48. A) Moderate variability is present

Bradycardia is nonhypoxic when moderate variability is present. Moderate variability has a high correlation with the absence of significant acidemia. A fetal heart rate baseline above 100 bpm is not necessarily associated with the absence of fetal hypoxia, especially if the variability is absent or marked. An absence of uterine activity is inconsequential in discerning whether a fetus experiencing bradycardia is hypoxic unless tachysystole or prolonged decelerations are present.

49. C) Place the patient in a lateral position

A chronic decrease in blood flow across the uteroplacental unit can result in fetal heart rate bradycardia. To improve placental perfusion, the nurse will place the patient in a lateral position. Vibroacoustic stimulation is not an appropriate intervention to improve uteroplacental blood flow. There is no indication the patient requires a vaginal examination; the nursing interventions should be focused on improving blood flow to the placenta.

50. C) Sinusoidal

This fetal heart rate (FHR) tracing denotes a pathologic sinusoidal pattern, which reflects smooth or almost smooth sine waveforms. They may have decelerations, but not accelerations. The pattern is not indeterminate because there is a clear recording of it on the tracing. A pseudo-sinusoidal pattern is characterized by periods of a normal FHR baseline, baseline variability, and other elements such as decelerations and accelerations.

51. C) Variability

On occasion, the fetal heart rate (FHR) baseline may be less than 110 bpm but also have reassuring signs such as moderate variability. The FHR variability is associated with fetal well-being. Moderate variably reflects adequate fetal oxygenation and is one of the most important predictive aspects of the FHR tracing. Neither the stage of labor nor the gestational age is correlated with fetal well-being or a baseline of 105 bpm.

52. C) Is referenced to atmospheric pressure

The intrauterine pressure catheter provides an absolute measurement of intra-amniotic pressure because it is referenced to atmospheric pressure or "zeroed." This capability allows for absolute measurement of intra-amniotic pressure. The fluid-filled sensor tip allows for measurement because the catheter can be referenced to atmospheric pressure. The sensor that detects myometrial tone is in a tocotransducer, not an intrauterine pressure catheter.

53. A) Exclude FHR accelerations

When determining the fetal heart rate (FHR) baseline, the nurse will approximate the mean FHR by rounding it to increments of 5 bpm during a 10-minute window. Accelerations and decelerations and periods of marked FHR variability are not considered when calculating an approximation of the FHR baseline.

54. A) 105 bpm

The fetal heart rate (FHR) baseline the nurse should associate with the report is 105 bpm, which is bradycardic. Bradycardia is defined as a baseline below 110 bpm. An FHR of 115 and 125 bpm is within the acceptable range of 110 to 160 bpm.

55. A) The patient who smokes

The nicotine in a cigarette constricts the blood vessels in the placenta, decreasing oxygenated blood flow to the fetus. Multiple gestations do not cause diminished placental function and is not a medical condition. Cervical incompetence refers to a cervix that dilates early, resulting in the loss of a fetus or premature birth.

56. B) Prolonged

Tachysystole can cause prolonged or late decelerations. Prolonged decelerations can occur because the uteroplacental blood flow is diminished. Early decelerations are caused by vagal stimulation, not tachysystole. Variable decelerations are caused by compression of the umbilical cord, not tachysystole.

57. B) Glucose is broken down

The normal fetal metabolic process begins as glucose is broken down into lactic acid. Carbon dioxide is a waste product of the fetal metabolic process and is removed by diffusion across the placenta. Oxygen is required to facilitate the conversion of lactic acid into carbon dioxide and water, but the delivery of oxygen to the fetus is not the beginning of the metabolic process.

58. B) Ultrasound

If repetitive variable decelerations are present, the nurse will anticipate preparing the patient for an ultrasound to evaluate the amniotic fluid volume. Oligohydramnios is an underlying cause of the pattern and is associated with increased perinatal morbidity and mortality. A contraction stress test can increase the chance of fetal hypoxia because the uterine contractions impede uteroplacental blood flow. A vibroacoustic stimulator is used to elicit fetal accelerations and is not an appropriate intervention for this patient.

59. C) There may be a discrepancy between the monitor and strip chart

There may be a discrepancy between a fetal heart rate tracing on a central monitor display and the bedside strip chart. The dimensions of a strip chart displayed on a computer screen may vary from the original strip chart at the bedside. Therefore, the information is not always very accurate, nor does the strip chart at the bedside look completely different.

60. B) Five

Three to five uterine contractions within 10 minutes is considered a normal pattern. Four contractions in 10 minutes are not the maximum number of contractions in a normal pattern. Six contractions in 10 minutes averaged over a period of 30 minutes is considered tachysystole.

61. B) Indeterminate variable

The decelerations occurring are variable, and the nurse will document the decelerations as indeterminate because the uterine contraction pattern cannot be interpreted. Periodic and episodic changes refer to changes in the fetal heart rate (FHR) that occur in response to contractions. The description of the changes in the FHR is not late or early decelerations; they are variable.

62. C) Requires further patient evaluation

Marked variability can be caused by fetal activity or stimulation and can also signify that the fetus may be mildly hypoxic or hemodynamically compromised. Therefore, the nurse must further evaluate the patient when considering the clinical causation of the finding. Marked variability is not a reassuring sign.

63. B) Discontinue the oxytocin

The nurse will discontinue the oxytocin as part of initiating uterine resuscitation measures. A patient with a category II tracing with absent fetal heart rate (FHR) accelerations and minimal FHR variability requires intrauterine resuscitation measures. Continuing to monitor the patient increases the risk of fetal compromise. Delivery is unnecessary unless the tracing progresses to a category III, which includes absent variability and repetitive late or variable decelerations.

64. B) Fetal trophoblast

The fetal trophoblast in the placenta serves as a filter, permitting the maternal–fetal exchange of nutrients and waste products and preventing maternal–fetal blood exchange. The placenta transfers oxygen and nutrients and removes waste products through the chorionic villi, which are then filtered by the fetal trophoblast. Blood enters the intervillous space under positive arterial pressure, bathes the fetal villi, and then drains back to the maternal veins.

65. A) Mild cord compression

The presence of uniform accelerations is usually in response to either mild cord compression or a breech presentation. It is a benign pattern. Uniform accelerations are not associated with the second stage of labor or uteroplacental insufficiency.

66. C) Recurrent variable decelerations

Recurrent variable decelerations with absent variability meet the criteria for a category III tracing, which is considered abnormal. Fetal bradycardia, not tachycardia in the presence of absent variability, reflects a category III tracing. A pseudo-sinusoidal pattern is a temporary fetal heart rate pattern that can appear when the patient receives an opioid narcotic in labor and is a benign pattern.

67. B) 15 seconds

The term acceleration for a fetus greater than 32 weeks' gestation refers to a transient increase in the amplitude of 15 beats or greater above the fetal heart rate baseline for at least 15 seconds in duration. A duration of 10 seconds is insufficient. A duration of 20 seconds exceeds the minimum requirement.

68. A) Epidural analgesia

Uterine tachysystole can be caused by many factors and can adversely affect the oxygenation of the fetus. An epidural is a factor associated with the development of tachysystole. Fetal movement and maternal hypotension are not associated with the development of tachysystole.

69. B) Patient safety issue

Nursing staff competency must be regularly validated to ensure patient safety and quality of care. A 3-year lapse in validation is a patient safety issue. An ethical dilemma refers to a situation in which a difficult choice must be made between two courses of action, either of which entails transgressing a moral principle. Quality improvement is a process used to improve clinical practice.

70. C) Immediately before

The most optimal time to evaluate the fetal heart rate (FHR) baseline in a laboring patient is in the period immediately prior to the onset of a uterine contraction because it is most likely to be discernable. During and immediately after a uterine contraction is the most likely time when periodic changes in the FHR occur. The FHR baseline is not evaluated during periodic changes.

71. C) Sinusoidal pattern

A sinusoidal pattern is associated with placental abruption. Early decelerations result from compression of the fetal head during a contraction that stimulates the parasympathetic system. Early decelerations are not pathologic. Prolonged accelerations are not a finding associated with a sinusoidal pattern. Prolonged accelerations are accelerations that last at least 2 minutes but continue for less than 10 minutes and are reassuring.

72. B) Rhythm

Most fetal dysrhythmias are recognizable on a strip chart as abrupt changes in the rhythm or rates between beats (RR interval) of the fetal heart rate (FHR). The FHR baseline and variability are affected by the specific type of fetal dysrhythmia.

73. **C) Reposition the patient**

Maternal repositioning, more specifically ensuring the supine position is avoided while also promoting right or left lateral positioning, is the correct response. Lateral positioning has been shown to optimize fetal hemoglobin saturation levels while also enabling fetal position changes, which can relieve the pressure on the umbilical cord. Continuing to observe the patient is a component of variable deceleration management, but not the first action needed to be taken. While decreasing or discontinuing oxytocin may be a piece of deceleration management, it is not the first intervention with variable decelerations.

74. **A) Affirming the presence of a fetal heart rate with a handheld Doppler**

Preterm fetuses can be a challenge to monitor, which requires the nurse to evaluate the type, value, and quality of information obtained. When monitoring an extremely preterm fetus, the nurse will consider affirming the presence of a fetal heart rate with a handheld Doppler due to the difficulty obtaining a tracing. Planning to continuously adjust an external monitor or applying the external monitor to the middle of the abdomen are not effective actions with an extremely preterm fetus.

75. **A) Either the fetal vertex or breech**

The fetal heart rate responses and movement are identical regardless of vibroacoustic stimulation application to the fetal breech or vertex.

76. **C) Three to five contractions every 10 minutes**

Normal uterine activity is defined as a frequency of three to five contractions in 10 minutes with a strength of 25 to 75 mmHg and a duration of 60 to 90 seconds. Contraction strength of 80 to 100 mmHg and duration of 90 to 120 seconds can result in fetal retention of carbon dioxide.

77. **C) Minimal**

The type of variability the nurse can anticipate for a fetus that is 27 weeks' gestation is minimal. The autonomic nervous system of a fetus less than 32 weeks' gestation is not fully developed, reflected by less variability. Absent or marked variability are not fetal heart rate findings associated with a fetus at 27 weeks' gestation. Absent variability is associated with fetal hypoxia or acidosis, and marked variability can be associated with fetal movement, activity, or hypoxia.

78. **B) Determines the pH**

The balance of hydrogen (H^+) and hydroxyl (OH^-) ions determines the degree of acidity and alkalinity, which make up the pH. Carbon dioxide is a waste product of the breakdown of lactic acid. The level of the partial pressure of carbon dioxide ($PaCO_2$) is associated with the oxygen content of the fetal blood and the ability to eliminate the $PaCO_2$. The pH does not directly affect fetal oxygenation. Fetal oxygenation and the $PaCO_2$ have an inverse relationship.

79. **A) Decreased fetal movement**

It is important for the nurse to understand the physiology of a fetus experiencing acidosis. When a fetus is unable to excrete nonvolatile acid in utero, the nurse can anticipate a decrease in or lack of fetal movement, absent fetal tone, and loss of fetal breathing movements.

80. C) Within 30 minutes

The recommended time is 30 minutes from decision to incision. The support person's absence should not have any effect on the timing of a Cesarean section being done regarding fetal well-being. It is ideal to perform the procedure as soon as possible, but a quantifiable time frame is needed.

81. B) 155 bpm

The fetal heart rate (FHR) baseline is determined by approximating the mean FHR rounded up to increments of 5 bpm during a 10-minute window. This approximation excludes accelerations and decelerations, and periods of marked FHR variability. If the FHR baseline is plotted over a visually wider range such as 20 minutes, it may be helpful to calculate the mean and then round off. The bulk of the FHR baseline data is plotted on the fetal strip chart between 146 and 160 bpm; the mean FHR would be calculated by adding these two integers (146 + 160) and dividing the result by 2 (306 ÷ 2). The mean (in this case, 153) would then be rounded to the nearest increment of 5. Therefore, the correct result is 155 bpm. The FHR rates of 150 and 160 bpm are incorrect estimations.

82. C) Instruct the patient to return to the clinic in a week

The nurse will instruct the patient to return to the clinic in a week. Between 28 and 32 weeks' gestation, there is only a small chance that the nonstress test will be reactive. The fetal autonomic nervous system may not have reached the maturity necessary to elicit the fetal heart rate criteria of 10 beats above the baseline for 10 seconds that a fetus at 32 weeks' gestation should. Although medications, nutrition, and hydration can affect the fetus, these factors cannot be attributed to the fact that the autonomic nervous system is immature.

83. C) Reposition the patient

Periodic variable decelerations occur because of compression or occlusion of the umbilical cord. Transient compression of the umbilical cord is usually corrected by altering the maternal position. Scalp stimulation is performed when there is a concern about the possibility of fetal acidosis. Administering oxygen to the patient will not alleviate the periodic cord compression.

84. A) Activate the chain of command

The nurse is legally and ethically responsible for the safety of the patient. A patient with a non reassuring tracing should not be discharged home; therefore, the nurse will activate the chain of command. If there is a difference of opinion between the nurse and healthcare provider regarding the interventions and plan of care for a patient, the nurse should activate the chain of command to obtain a resolution to the situation. Discharging the patient places the patient and fetus at risk for injury or death. The ethics committee is used when an ethical issue arises or an issue is unresolved; this does not include clinical decisions that require an expert in the specific area of practice, such as fetal monitor interpretation.

85. B) Polyhydramnios

Iatrogenic polyhydramnios is a concern during an amnioinfusion and should be monitored by evaluating the intake and output of fluid being administered. Iatrogenic oligohydramnios is not associated with amnioinfusion. Oligohydramnios refers to decreased amniotic fluid. An amnioinfusion is performed to instill fluid into the uterine cavity. Iatrogenic tachysystole is not a complication of an amnioinfusion. The administration of oxytocin can cause tachysystole.

86. C) A patient with type 1 diabetes in spontaneous labor

Type 1 diabetes affects the development and functioning of the placenta, increasing the risk of utero-placental insufficiency. Late fetal heart rate deceleration reflects uteroplacental insufficiency. A patient at 34 weeks' gestation in premature labor is not at risk for uteroplacental insufficiency; therefore, late decelerations are not anticipated. Nalbuphine is an opioid analgesic administered for pain and is not generally associated with uteroplacental insufficiency.

87. B) Responses

The final step in interpreting a fetal heart rate (FHR) tracing is to assess for changes that may occur in response to contractions, referred to as periodic changes, and those that occur intermittently, referred to as episodic changes. Assessing the FHR baseline is the first step, followed by the assessment of the variability.

88. A) Marked variability

Marked variability is defined as fluctuations in the fetal heart rate (FHR) baseline of more than 25 bpm. The significance of a heart rate with such pronounced beat-to-beat range is uncertain. Assessing an FHR pattern with such a wide variance in bpm prevents an accurate interpretation of baseline rate. Moderate variability is defined as having an amplitude that ranges between 6 and 25 bpm. It is associated with autonomic regulation of the FHR not affected by any interruption in oxygenation. Minimal variability is defined as an amplitude range that is detectable but equal to or less than 5 bpm. This range of variability can be associated with problems such as fetal metabolic acidemia or preexisting neurologic injuries as well as benign circumstances like fetal sleep cycles.

89. C) Place the patient in a lateral position

Late decelerations reflect the fetal response to hypoxemia resulting from maternal, fetal, or placental conditions that impede fetal oxygenation. Therefore, the nurse will reposition the patient laterally to improve maternal blood flow to the placenta. There is no indication that a cervical examination is necessary; the nurse's priority is to improve maternal–fetal oxygenation. Continuing to monitor the patient will not improve maternal–fetal oxygenation.

90. C) It is a recognized tool to validate competency

Regulatory agencies such as The Joint Commission accept a written exam as a method of evidence that an institution has made an appropriate effort to validate competency. Exam writers should be educated on the rigorous process of test item writing for the exam to be a valid assessment. Exams are generally targeted to one type of clinician, making them an insular activity that is not useful to assess the competency of multiple disciplines.

91. A) Absent

Because the amplitude range of the fetal heart rate (FHR) is undetectable, it is referred to as absent. Moderate variability refers to fluctuations in the FHR baseline of 6 to 25 bpm. Marked variability refers to changes in the FHR baseline greater than 25 bpm.

92. C) Fetal tone

If both parameters of a modified biophysical profile (BPP) are reassuring, it can be assumed that the result is equivalent to an 8/10. The conclusion assumes that if the nonstress test is reactive, fetal tone and movement are likely present. A BPP is not an antepartum assessment for fetal growth. A score of 8/10 for a modified BPP is not an assumption that fetal breathing is present.

93. B) 10

Because the autonomic nervous system of a fetus may not be fully developed at 31 weeks' gestation, the nurse can anticipate the fetal heart rate (FHR) beats above the baseline to be 10 beats. The overall criteria that are a predictor of fetal well-being for a fetus less than 32 weeks' gestation is a transient increase of 10 or more beats above the baseline sustained for at least 10 seconds. The fetus should have an increase of greater than 5 beats above the baseline. Some fetuses below 32 weeks may exhibit an FHR pattern with 15 beats above the baseline for 15 or more seconds; if this is the case, the fetus should continue to meet this criterion during any additional periods of monitoring.

94. B) Discontinue monitoring the patient

The nurse will discontinue monitoring the patient. Because the fetus is less than 28 weeks' gestation, the nurse will not anticipate seeing any accelerations; however, the baseline variability indicates the fetus is well oxygenated. A biophysical profile will not be performed because the fetus is extremely premature.

95. B) Minimal

Minimal or absent variability is often associated with patterns of fetal dysrhythmia. Moderate and marked variability is not commonly noted because there is a disruption in the conduction of the cardiac signal.

96. C) Resolving variable decelerations

Amnioinfusion is indicated for managing variable decelerations and acts by creating a cushion of fluid that protects the umbilical cord from compression. Studies have shown that amnioinfusion is not effective in preventing meconium aspiration syndrome or perinatal death. Amnioinfusion does not delay active labor or affect the length of labor.

97. A) Implement acoustic stimulation

Using acoustic stimulation is an appropriate action to shorten the testing time for a biophysical profile (BPP), specifically the nonstress test (NST) component. Omitting the NST is not appropriate because it is a primary component of both a BPP and a modified BPP. A contraction stress test will not reduce the testing time and is not a component of a BPP.

98. A) Fetal hypoxia

Late decelerations occur when the fetus is hypoxic. A fetal sleep pattern is associated with decreased variability, not late decelerations. Umbilical cord compression results in variable decelerations.

99. C) Uterine activity

During labor, the fetal heart rate (FHR) is analyzed in relation to uterine activity. The stress of the uterine contractions and the resulting FHR pattern are indicators of fetal well-being. Fetal movement is not a factor considered with the FHR. A biophysical profile is not routinely performed during labor.

100. C) Loss of fetal heart rate activity

The first change be noted for a fetus with hypoxia will be on a nonstress test. A loss of fetal heart rate activity will occur with fetal hypoxia. The loss of fetal heart rate activity is followed by decreased fetal breathing movements, then a decrease in amniotic fluid, and finally a loss of fetal movement, then tone.

101. A) Auscultate the FHR with a handheld Doppler

When a fetal scalp electrode (FSE) is used to obtain a fetal heart rate (FHR) tracing, interference with the signal can occur. Auscultation of the FHR with a handheld Doppler can provide information about the FHR and rhythm. Using an external fetal monitor is not a reliable method for differentiating between artifact and dysrhythmia because the signal may not get recorded correctly. Performing a vaginal examination to determine the placement of the FSE does not allow the nurse to differentiate between artifact and dysrhythmia.

102. B) Minimal

The variability of the tracing is minimal. Minimal variability has a fluctuation of the baseline of 5 beats or less a minute. Marked variability refers to a fluctuation in the fetal heart rate (FHR) of more than 25 beats a minute. Moderate variability refers to fluctuations in the FHR of 6 to 25 beats a minute.

103. A) Alloimmunization

A risk of blood type incompatibility between mother and fetus during an amniocentesis is alloimmunization. Infection and bleeding are risk factors for any amniocentesis, regardless of blood type compatibility. Maternal/fetal blood type incompatibility is responsible for conditions like hydrops fetalis that can lead to fetal death.

104. C) Transient fetal head compression

The transient fetal head compression associated with uterine contractions can often be seen with a fetus that is engaged in the maternal pelvis. Pressure that is exerted against the fetal head in turn affects fetal intracranial pressure and/or cerebral blood flow. This, in turn, triggers the parasympathetic system, which causes the gradual slowing of the fetal heart rate (FHR). Once this pressure is relieved, autonomic reflexes subside with a return to FHR baseline. Early decelerations are not associated with a disruption of oxygenation. Maternal administration of narcotics does not cause early decelerations.

105. B) Averaged after 30 minutes

Uterine activity is quantified by counting the number of contractions that occur in a 10-minute period and then averaging that number after 30 minutes. Uterine activity is calculated from the average. The average is calculated after 30 minutes based on three 10-minute windows.

106. B) "Nurses implement independent interventions."
It is within the scope of practice for the RN to implement independent interventions in response to the fetal heart rate (FHR) changes within the context of the clinical assessment. Interventions in response to FHR changes within the context of the clinical assessment are not dependent. The support of independent interventions in response to FHR changes is reflected in the institutional interprofessional policies and guidelines, not the Nurse Practice Act.

107. A) A G1P0 patient who has had a nonreactive nonstress test for over 20 minutes
Scalp stimulation is only performed during labor after cervical dilatation has occurred. Based on the different patient data, scalp stimulation would be appropriate for the patient with a nonreactive nonstress test after 20 minutes. There is no contraindication to scalp stimulation on twin gestations during labor.

108. B) Normal acid–base balance
The umbilical cord arterial gas reflects a normal acid–base balance. The anticipated range of an arterial cord sample is a pH of 7.18 to 7.38, PO_2 of 5.6 to 30.8 mmHg, $PaCO_2$ of 32.2 to 65.8 mmHg, and a base excess of 0 to 11 mEq/L. The results of the arterial cord blood sample do not correlate with metabolic acidosis or respiratory acidosis.

109. A) Chorioamnionitis
A fetal heart rate (FHR) baseline above 160 bpm is considered tachycardic. Chorioamnionitis is an intra-amniotic infection for which the nurse can anticipate fetal tachycardia. Fetal hypothermia results in fetal bradycardia, and is indicated by an FHR baseline of less than 110 bpm for at least 10 minutes. When an electrical impulse reenters the ventricle, the fetus may experience supraventricular tachycardia.

110. C) Not reducing the overall Cesarean section rate and being exceedingly difficult to place
The two most significant drawbacks of fetal pulse oximetry are the difficulty with the physical placement of the probe and the failure to reduce the overall Cesarean section birth rate. High cost was not associated with fetal pulse oximetry, nor was it found to be highly accurate. Difficulty distinguishing between maternal and fetal oxygenation was not a driving factor in the abandonment of this technology.

111. C) Constantly maintains maximum dilation
The uterine vascular bed constantly maintains maximum dilatation. The placental vessels are not controlled by the central nervous system or level of fetal oxygenation.

112. A) Palpate the maternal pulse and compare it to the audible signal
If there is ever any concern about the maternal heart rate being recorded on a fetal heart rate (FHR) tracing, the nurse can quickly palpate the maternal pulse and compare it to the audible signal. It is unnecessary to apply a fetal scalp electrode (FSE) to distinguish between the maternal heart rate and FHR. The application of an FSE is invasive. Performing Leopold's maneuver and reapplying the external monitor does not help the nurse distinguish between a maternal heart rate and FHR. It provides information about the position of the fetus and helps locate the correct area on the maternal abdomen to place an external monitor.

113.   A) Fetal bradycardia

The tracing denotes bradycardia of a term fetus with a stable baseline rate between 100 and 110 bpm prior to delivery. Bradycardia is a fetal heart rate that is below 120 bpm if the fetus is preterm and below 110 bpm if the fetus is term. A bradycardic rate is sustained for 10 or more minutes. The variability in this tracing is minimal. The tracing is not indeterminate.

114.   A) Antiarrhythmic

Supraventricular tachycardia is characterized by a fetal heart rate baseline of 200 bpm and requires an intervention to treat the pattern. A common intervention is the administration of an antiarrhythmic. A beta-blocker is not administered for supraventricular tachycardia. Beta-blockers are used to treat arrhythmias such as atrial fibrillation. Atropine is not administered for supraventricular tachycardia. Atropine is used to treat bradycardia.

115.   B) 37 weeks' gestation with decreased fetal movement

A woman at 37 weeks' gestation presenting with decreased fetal movement is an appropriate candidate for a contraction stress test (CST). A CST should not be performed on women if it would pose a maternal or fetal risk. A woman with a previous Cesarean section is at risk for uterine rupture, and a 34-week gestation fetus is preterm.

116.   C) Promotes evidence-based practice

Because guidelines and standards of care for a medical record audit are used as a framework for validating competence, a medical record audit can serve as an opportunity to promote evidence-based practice and streamline clinical care. Medical record audits are beneficial for both new and experienced nurses. They can be used for competence validation providing data regarding a requisite knowledge base and the essential clinical skills necessary for intrapartum practice. An orientation checklist is most beneficial to ensure that all skills are covered during orientation.

117.   A) Above

A fetal heart rate baseline of 165 bpm is above the normal parameters of 110 to 160 bpm and is referred to as fetal tachycardia. A baseline below 110 bpm, referred to as bradycardia, is below the acceptable parameters.

118.   B) Audit the nurse's medical records

The educator will randomly select medical records and external fetal monitoring strips to audit and review with the nurse. This can be used as both a learning exercise and as part of the validation of competency. This exercise can identify the strengths of the nurse and areas in which the nurse requires further orientation. Reviewing the orientation checklist or administering a fetal heart rate pattern interpretation exam does not provide the depth of information gained from a medical record audit.

119.   C) Maternal intake of caffeine

Isolated extrasystoles occur as a result of premature atrial contractions (PACs) and premature ventricular contractions (PVCs). Both conditions are commonly caused by maternal intake of caffeine. A fetal sleep cycle is not associated with isolated extrasystoles; however, the variability can be decreased during a fetal sleep cycle. An abnormal fetal presentation is not associated with the development of PACs or PVCs, nor it is associated with isolated extrasystoles. PACs and PVCs are associated with changes in the electrical conductivity of the cardiac system.

120. A) Exchange of maternal–fetal blood cells

When villi break off within the intervillous space, maternal and fetal blood cells are exchanged. Fetal hyperglycemia occurs when maternal glucose levels are significantly elevated. Maternal immunoglobulins are not transferred to the fetus when the villi break off within the intervillous space; the maternal and fetal blood cells are exchanged.

121. C) The strength of the contractions

Montevideo units are calculated by evaluating the strength of a uterine contraction and resting period. This information is recorded on the tracing and reflected in millimeters of mercury (mmHg). The frequency and duration of the contractions are not reflected in mmHg; they are reflected in seconds and minutes and are not included in the calculation of Montevideo units.

122. C) Turn off the oxytocin

A normal uterine contraction pattern refers to three to five contractions in 10 minutes. A patient who, over the past 30 minutes, averages seven contractions in a 10-minute period is experiencing tachysystole. Tachysystole can result in inadequate oxygenation to the fetus; therefore, the nurse should turn off the oxytocin to help resolve the tachysystole. Increasing the intravenous fluid and repositioning the patient laterally are intrauterine resuscitation measures to facilitate the delivery of oxygenated blood to the fetus. However, there is no indication the fetus requires these interventions, and these interventions will not help decrease the uterine activity.

123. A) Buffer system is activated

When aerobic metabolism is no longer effective, lactic acid builds up, causing retention of hydrogen ions; an increase in their presence in the blood results in acidemia and an increase in the tissues causes acidosis. These changes activate the fetal buffer system to reduce acidosis. When aerobic metabolism occurs, the fetal pH decreases due to the buildup of lactic acid. The fetal demand for oxygen increases to help restore homeostasis.

124. B) The CST is an earlier predictor of a deteriorating fetal status than a nonstress test

The contraction stress test (CST) is used to observe the fetal heart rate response to three palpable contractions and is an earlier predictor of a deteriorating fetal status than a nonstress test. The CST carries a high false-positive rate, meaning the late decelerations are present during testing, but the fetus is tolerant of subsequent labor induction. When the CST is reassuring, the risk of fetal death within 7 days is minimal.

125. B) Pseudo-sinusoidal

The pattern reflects a pseudo-sinusoidal pattern, which will have periods of a normal fetal heart rate (FHR) baseline, baseline variability, and other elements such as spontaneous or induced accelerations. A pseudo-sinusoidal pattern reflects a responsive heart and neurologic system when the fetus is relaxed and may be making small movement in utero. A sinusoidal pattern refers to an FHR baseline with an undulating pattern, repetitively creating a constant sine waveform.

POP QUIZ ANSWERS

CHAPTER 2
POP QUIZ 2.1

The best way to improve uteroplacental circulation is to stabilize maternal–fetal oxygen status. To stabilize maternal–fetal oxygen status, the nurse should change the position of the patient, administer an IV fluid bolus, and administer supplemental oxygen as needed.

CHAPTER 3
POP QUIZ 3.1

The nurse should call the provider to the bedside.

POP QUIZ 3.2

The amniotic sac must be broken, which means there is an increased risk of infection.

POP QUIZ 3.3

Uterine tachysystole is defined as more than five contractions in 10 minutes.

POP QUIZ 3.4

The fetus may be in a sleep cycle. Vibroacoustic stimulation can be performed to attempt to wake the fetus out of the sleep cycle.

POP QUIZ 3.5

It is not normal. It is normal for *decelerations* to occur with pushing. The nurse should continue to monitor the fetus and also monitor the patient's pulse. If there still appear to be fetal accelerations, a fetal scalp electrode may be requested.

CHAPTER 4
POP QUIZ 4.1

The nurse should change the patient's position, administer an IV fluid bolus, administer oxygen 8 to 10 L per nonrebreather mask, and call the provider. *Note:* Per institutional guidelines, the IV fluid bolus will be lactated Ringer's solution or normal saline.

POP QUIZ 4.2

Variability is the most important characteristic of fetal heart rate tracings in determining fetal well-being.

POP QUIZ 4.3

Variable decelerations may be resolved with amnioinfusion due to the decrease of cord compression.

CHAPTER 5

POP QUIZ 5.1

The concern for this patient would be at the maternal circulation step of the maternal–fetal oxygenation pathway. An interruption here can cause decreased cardiac output, altering fetal oxygenation.

POP QUIZ 5.2

Eclampsia is a possible diagnosis.

POP QUIZ 5.3

The nurse is attempting to prevent pulmonary edema.

POP QUIZ 5.4

The nurse could mention signs of preeclampsia (such as headache, blurred vision, epigastric pain, and swelling), eclampsia (seizures), or HELLP syndrome (abdominal pain).

POP QUIZ 5.5

The risk is for compression of the inferior vena cava, which can cause hypotension, late decelerations in the fetus, and possibly fetal death.

POP QUIZ 5.6

First, the nurse should call for help. Then, the nurse should insert a straight or Foley catheter into the bladder. It is likely that the bladder is filling or full and is displacing the uterus, causing the excessive bleeding.

POP QUIZ 5.7

The patient is likely experiencing an abruptio placentae. The nurse should call for help and a provider. The nurse should then prepare for an emergent cesarean section with full neonatal resuscitation. A urine drug screen (suspected cocaine) and a blood transfusion may be ordered.

POP QUIZ 5.8

The nurse should prepare for a possible shoulder dystocia by having extra nurses at the delivery, including one to care for the neonate. A stool should be available on each side of the bed in case suprapubic pressure is needed. A nurse should be assigned to document what happens at delivery.

CHAPTER 6

POP QUIZ 6.1

Respect for patient autonomy applies in this case. The nurse may feel that they do not have time to follow this evidence-based practice, but the patient has a right to it as long as the neonate is stable.

POP QUIZ 6.2

The principle of justice applies because the nurse is helping to ensure that underserved patients also receive adequate care.

POP QUIZ 6.3

The nurse must use the chain of command as determined by institutional policy. This means a call should be made to the next person in charge, and the nurse may need to go beyond that person if there is no response.

POP QUIZ 6.4

The nurse did not follow standard of care and could face legal action.

POP QUIZ 6.5

This is an example of debriefing.

POP QUIZ 6.6

The process is called PDSA (plan, do, study, act).

INDEX

Page entries that appear in italics refer to content in the practice test and practice test answer chapters.